The Defense Rests
Lessons Learned Through Illness and Grief

The Defense Rests
Lessons Learned Through Illness and Grief

Kathryn Cosper

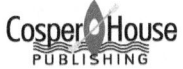

Copyright © 2020 by Kathryn P. Cosper

All rights reserved. No part of this book may be reproduced or transmitted in any form or by any means, electronic or mechanical, including photocopying, recording, or by any information storage and retrieval system, without the written permission of the author, except in the case of brief quotes in critical articles and reviews. For permission, contact the author at kathryncosper.com. Scripture quotations taken from the HOLY BIBLE, NEW INTERNATIONAL VERSION, Copyright (c) 1973,1978, 1984 by International Bible Society. Used by permission of Zondervan Publishing House.

Events, locales, occurrences, and conversations are recorded from the author's memories and from actual correspondence sent and received, including email and Facebook messages. Other than family members, no individuals in this story are identified by name.

ISBN: 978-1-7329958-6-4 (paperback)
ISBN: 978-1-7329958-8-8 (ebook)

Public Library catalogue data: Branch call number 305.908709 (Cosper)

Cover and interior designs: Diana Wade
Cover and inside photography: Kathryn P. Cosper
First edition February 2020
Second edition August 2020
Charlotte, North Carolina
www.kathryncosper.com

Printed in the United States of America

for Harvey

*My day is done, and I am like a boat
drawn on the beach, listening to the dance-music
of the tide in the evening.*

Rabindranath Tagore,
The Heart of God

Contents

Why I Wrote This Book		5
Our Life Before		11
Part 1	**When Illness Is New**	**17**
Chapter 1	Becoming a Patient	19
Chapter 2	When a Loved One Becomes a Patient	43
Chapter 3	When a Friend Becomes Ill	69
Chapter 4	Ways to Say We Care	95
Chapter 5	Rehabilitation	107
Part 2	**When Illness Becomes Disability**	**123**
Chapter 6	When Home Is Not the Same, Episode 1	125
Chapter 7	Another Chance to Prepare for Home	139
Chapter 8	Life Goes On, Even When It Changes	163
Chapter 9	When Home is Not the Same, Episode 2	187
Chapter 10	When a New Normal Never Comes	201
Chapter 11	The Goodbyes Begin	215
Part 3	**When Illness Divides the Home**	**231**
Chapter 12	Losing Our Options	233
Chapter 13	The End of Living Together	247
Chapter 14	Long-Term Care, Short-Term	263
Chapter 15	Redefining Hope	281
Part 4	**When a Loved One Dies**	**289**
Chapter 16	Mourning and Grief	291
Chapter 17	Words for Expressing Sympathy	313
Chapter 18	The Goodbyes Continue	325
Part 5	**When Life Goes On**	**335**
Chapter 19	Living With Grief	337
Chapter 20	A Widow Writes to Her Husband	347
Chapter 21	The Time After	359
Acknowledgments		371
Suggested Reading		375

Why I Wrote This Book

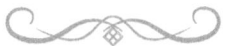

Many of us are living pretty ordinary lives, busy with families, friends, jobs, and activities, when, suddenly or over time, one of us becomes seriously ill.

We are new at being patients, or we are new at being the family members, caregivers, and friends of patients. No one has taught us how to fill these unwelcome roles, so we have to learn as we go. We are surprised by how little control we have over what is happening, and we are overwhelmed by the decisions we face in what we can control. We don't always know what to say or do, and we are frustrated by our inability to "fix" things—for ourselves or for the people we care about. The medical system is complex, the learning curve is steep, and sick persons need support in many ways.

Then, the unthinkable happens: a precious one dies. In a moment, our lives change forever. We are playing a part in a movie, but we don't know the script. We wander in deep sadness while the rest of the world is blithely moving on. Somehow we must find our way in a "new normal" life.

This book is the story of a man and his family as they struggled through his illness and, eventually, his death. It is the story of a wife who was unprepared for the challenges they faced and of the lessons she learned. It is the story of a family who supported one another and of people known and unknown who helped them along the way.

Every person, every story is different. Our ways of handling our struggles are as individual as our fingerprints. But each of us knows people who are ill. Each of us will eventually be a player in the drama of serious illness and death.

At the urging of friends, I first attempted to write a book about the illness and death of my husband, Harvey, as a context in which to share ideas about how to help people going through such difficult times. It was not supposed to be about me. But that first draft turned out to be merely a long series of happenings and suggestions—and, while I was narrating them, I was hiding behind them. I was the practical, it-is-what-it-is person, the get-on-with-it person, the reporter of straight news. Interpreting those happenings, becoming an honest character in the story, was not in my comfort zone. The story was hollow because it was not the whole truth.

So I traveled back into those hard years. It wasn't fun, and I cried a lot. Though I rejoiced in the moments of tenderness and genuine helpfulness, I recognized how far I had to go in acceptance and healing. I tried to grant myself patience and forgiveness for all of my failures and shortcomings throughout our ordeal. And I began to think about the shoes.

One morning, I had stepped into the elevator to visit Harvey during his fifth inpatient rehabilitation among nearly twenty hospitalizations in two years. Instead of my usual jeans or sweat

Why I Wrote This Book

pants, I had dressed up in a skirt and tights for a rare lunch away from the hospital with several friends. As she exited at her floor, a no-nonsense nurse looked over her shoulder at me with an eye roll and said, "You know about your shoes, right?" I looked down to see that I was wearing one plain, black, pointy-toed boot and one brown, square-toed boot with a gold buckle. When I arrived at Harvey's room, he remarked, "You have another set just like that at home."

Those shoes became a metaphor for the last years of my husband's life, when we lived in the tension between two very different places at the same time. Not just physical places, but spaces of contradictory realities and emotions: situations that were both pathetic and funny; that brought blessing out of misfortune, gratitude out of despair, comfort out of frustration, intimacy out of embarrassment, appreciation out of fear, grace out of confusion, and love out of mourning.

I became filled with compassion for our human selves. I realized that Harvey and I had made that long, hard walk together in the best way we could at the time. We traveled in mismatched shoes, but we were surrounded by grace. And, while I lost the person who was the love of my life, I had the love of my life.

Then I wrote the book that I wish I could have read before our hard times began.

What follows is a personal account of my husband's illness from autoimmune disorders, heart disease, and stroke; his disability over three years, and his death. It is the story of how we tried to deal with it all and how other people responded. It includes suggestions for patients, family members, caregivers, and friends in coping and helping during hard times. Though the perspective is that of a widow, many of the suggestions apply to the illness and death of other loved ones, as well.

We all see life through different lenses. In our family, we see through the lens of our Christian faith. Because Harvey had a successful career and excellent insurance, we see through the lens of financial security. Our forty-five-year marriage, with thriving children and grandchildren, created the lens of a stable home life. Having resided in the same area of the same city and been active in the same large church for forty years, we have had a strong, supportive social network. These are all advantages that so many others never have. All around us are people who experience trauma and tragedy too terrible to imagine and families who lack the financial and social resources to ease their heavy burdens. But in the end, the ugliness of illness, suffering, death, and grief is universal, and no amount of support or resources can take it away.

I do not pretend to speak on behalf of everyone who has experienced a stroke or heart disease, served as a caregiver for a disabled family member, or lost a loved one. I don't speak for all widows, Christians, or people who mourn. This is our family's story, and the suggestions come from our experience. Even so, I have read and listened to the stories of scores of people who have struggled through similar experiences, as well as counselors, pastors, and grief specialists, and I know there is much in our story that is shared by others. Although we can never presume to fully understand what another person is going through, our narratives build connection, and connection leads to understanding, and understanding engenders compassion. Sharing our stories can help us heal.

Our story unfolds through emails and Facebook updates to friends written over a period of five years, sprinkled within narrative from my perspective today. For easy access, within the story you will find practical suggestions and lessons we learned from our experience highlighted in either bold type or bulleted lists. I have included some messages we received from others, because they speak for themselves more strongly than any generalities I could give. I hope you will not find our humor inappropriate—that's just us. Where there are discrepancies between emails and narrative, you can tell that I was naïve about what was actually going on, or in denial, or trying to cheer our friends, family, and myself.

Were we lucky or unlucky? Feeling blessed or feeling sorry for ourselves? The answer: all of those. It is within that tension, in the world of contradictory realities, walking in our mismatched shoes through the bad and the good, that we have to live every day. It is there that we discover not just suffering and pain but also grace and love. It is there that God sends us where we need to be for those who need us, and it is there that God sends us exactly what we ourselves need. As God is gracious, so others are gracious to us, and so we can work at being gracious to others—kind, forbearing, and compassionate—forgiving ourselves when we fail.

I pray that telling our story will
- provide patients suffering through serious illness, their families, caregivers, and friends with helpful ideas on how to navigate the hard times;

- provide affirmation and comfort for those who are suffering illnesses and grieving the death of loved ones, assuring them that they are not alone;
- increase understanding and empathy for people who are sick and grieving, encouraging the ministry of presence in the lives of others; and
- promote the practice of gratitude, even in the hardest of times.

My purpose in writing this book is to inspire you to find, within yourself, your own best way to be a kind patient, a supportive spouse, an informed advocate, a caring friend.

Our Life Before

Harvey Lindenthal Cosper, Jr., and I met on a blind date at a fraternity party at the University of North Carolina at Chapel Hill in 1968. I was wearing a green wool sleeveless dress with covered buttons down the front; Harvey wore his gray flannel pants, white oxford-cloth button-down shirt with the sleeves rolled up, and brown loafers without socks. I was short, loud, and impulsive; he was tall, quiet, and deliberate. We each drove an old Chevy Corvair, that engineering marvel with the motor in the back. Our courtship was one of laughter and good friends, studying and dancing, music and cheap beer, parties and conversation, even during an era of unprecedented social change and political unrest.

During our final semester, while I was student teaching high school English in a nearby town, the university cancelled classes for days as students crowded onto the historic brick sidewalks that crossed the emerald grass under the giant old oaks of the main quad. Preppies and hippies marched together in protest of the United States' involvement in Vietnam and Cambodia, and members of the Black Student Movement took over a classroom building. But Harvey and I forged ahead with our own student lives. Shortly after graduation, he flew westward for five months of basic training as part of an Army Reserves medical unit.

On December 19, 1970, our friends and family joined us for a small wedding in the chapel of First Presbyterian Church in Greensboro, North Carolina, where I had spent my childhood. We began a good life together that would end on another December 19, many years into the future.

We didn't have much money, but we were happy. When Harvey's car died, we forked out five hundred dollars for an old red Volkswagen Beetle. As a marketing writer for an insurance company, I supported us on four hundred and ten dollars a month while Harvey, with some help for his tuition from his father, attended Wake Forest University School of Law. Despite careful planning, our first child was born early, during Harvey's final exams. After a few days in intensive care, the little guy we named Graham Harvey was able to come home to our gray four-room house near campus that we rented for eighty-five dollars a month. We later learned that "Graham" means "from the gray home."

After graduation, we moved to Charlotte for the remainder of our married life. Harvey practiced law, working more than fifty hours a week for many years. He built a reputation as a civil litigator specializing in medical malpractice defense. Meanwhile, I was a stay-at-home mom to three active children, a volunteer, singer, freelance writer, and part-time nonprofit employee with a "TAXIMOM" license plate. As with any growing family, there were the usual problems and issues. But, overall, we had a busy, cheerful life that sometimes reminded me of the "Leave It to

Beaver" and "Father Knows Best" families we had followed on our old black and white television when we were growing up in the fifties.

Every summer for years, we vacationed for ten days at one of North Carolina's beautiful beaches. Neighbors lined up to watch Harvey attach his little aluminum fishing boat, affectionately called "the Barnacle," to the back of our old station wagon, filling it with bicycles, strollers, coolers, fishing rods, tackle boxes, duffel bags, and a rusted gas grill. It might have been easier just to hook up the house and tow it on down the road. We sometimes talked of investing in our own place at the coast, maybe for retirement, long into the future.

A few days after our youngest child left for college, Harvey's stepmother called us to the hospital to say goodbye to his beloved father, a quirky, soft-spoken Southern gentleman and lawyer. After the funeral, Harvey surprised me by saying, "We've always loved the coast and wanted a place of our own there. I think we should go ahead and look into it. It would be an investment for the future that we could enjoy now. If we don't, it might never happen." Later, I remembered those prophetic words and wondered whether Harvey somehow sensed what was ahead for him.

We applied for a mortgage on a house in Wilmington, North Carolina, where, for a few days at a time over the next ten years, Harvey's ever-present briefcase detached from his arm and rarely left the back of the car. Many mornings, while I was still asleep, Harvey would awaken at dawn, slip into faded old clothes, and collect his favorite rods, lures, and bait along with a cooler from the garage. From the neighborhood marina, silhouetted against orange rays of sunlight spreading into the sky and reflecting in the Intracoastal Waterway, sipping from a thermos of coffee, he would glide through Masonboro Sound toward Wrightsville Beach or Carolina Beach, cruising the channels to reach the Atlantic Ocean in a small white fishing boat that he named the "Defense Rests." These peaceful outings reminded him of the many fishing trips he'd taken with his father over the years. He would return a few hours later to find me reading beside my dachshunds on the porch swing. He rarely snagged a fish big enough for lunch, but, for him, it wasn't just about the fishing.

In the years that followed, we visited the thin strip of Masonboro Island many times for walks and swims, and sometimes we were the only two people for as far as we could see. It was inhabited only by birds, turtles, crabs, and other small sea creatures moving amongst the dunes and scrub trees. On coastal visits, we weathered storms, kayaked, steamed oysters, and collected shells. Harvey used to joke that, when his time came to die, he was going to pack up the boat with a cooler of beer and a few cigars—and just drift to the east. I never foresaw that one day, all too soon, those sands and waters would welcome him for good.

In his mid-fifties, Harvey began to develop health issues and, by the age of sixty-four, he was suffering through one illness on top of another. Sickness and pain, surgeries and hospitalizations, the indignity of dependency and loss of privacy were difficult enough. Meanwhile, everyday life had to go on, with all of its complications. I became a sometimes clueless but always persistent helper. We did the only thing we could do: we got through one day at a time, with the help of many people.

Throughout it all, he remained a gentleman, and he rarely voiced a complaint. Harvey was an unusually humble man—especially for a trial lawyer. The only time he enjoyed being the center of attention was in the courtroom. Whenever anyone complimented him on his professional accomplishments, he replied that he was "just a plodder," simply getting up and working hard every day. But he was more than that: he worked with dedication, integrity, humor, and a spirit of calm. He modeled the belief that, no matter how contentious or uncomfortable a situation, even in adversarial relationships, we can always be civil and courteous to one another.

Though he disliked being the focus of attention, he was okay with the writing of this book; in fact, he suggested the idea while he was lying in intensive care for the first time. Having advocated for the medical profession over a thirty-eight-year career, he wanted to give some advice on how to be a good patient—which he absolutely was. He deflected attention from himself, and others could count on him for wise and generous words that often evoked smiles and laughter.

I do not mean to deify him here—he would hate that—although it is obvious the love and esteem accorded him by me and those who knew him. But his attitude of acceptance, his wry wit, his patience, and his determination to focus on others more than himself inspired and supported his family, friends, and co-workers during the difficult times as well as the good ones. He lived with a deep faith and a gratitude for life. He often referred to himself as "the luckiest man on the planet."

Harvey never made it to retirement at Masonboro Sound—not in the way he had hoped. He would not be walking our daughter down the aisle at her wedding or collecting baseballs with his grandchildren at major league parks. Those of us surviving him are grieving these losses now, for him and for ourselves. Yet we recognize, as he did, that we have been truly blessed by loving kindness and grace that helped carry us through all the difficult times we have faced.

I now believe that, in whatever circumstances we find ourselves, our highest calling as creatures made in the image of God is two-fold: to be grateful for the blessings of life and to demonstrate love for one another. Responding to this calling is so very difficult, and in our human frailty we often fail. But when we manage to live into this calling, we are able to find connection, purpose, and hope.

We cry together; and, in our pain, we help each other heal.

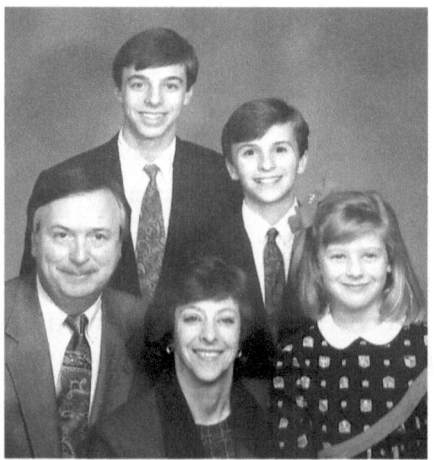

The family in earlier days

Part 1

When Illness Is New

The great thing, if one can, is to stop regarding all the unpleasant things as interruptions in one's 'own' or 'real' life. The truth is, of course, that what one calls interruptions are precisely one's real life – the life God is sending one day by day.
    C. S. Lewis, *The Collected Works of C.S. Lewis*

Chapter 1

Becoming a Patient

He is a wise man who does not grieve for the things which he has not, but rejoices for those which he has.

Epictetus

The Stroke

The Carolina blue sky was fading to dusk on that beautiful Saturday in April. Forty neighbors spilled from our house onto our back porch with drinks and tacos during a block party while I ran back upstairs to our bedroom to check on Harvey.

Earlier that day, we had been to Charlotte's Freedom Park for our grandson's Little League baseball game. Emerging from the car with a groan, Harvey trudged a short distance before stopping, hands on his knees, out of breath. He looked towards the field and wondered aloud whether he could make it across the grassy expanse to the bleachers as our son Graham strode over to offer his arm. Later, after the game, we joined Graham, his wife, Lisa, and our grandchildren for hot dogs and crispy onion rings.

Little did we suspect that would be Harvey's last meal for seventy days.

A busy sixty-four-year-old attorney, Harvey had been hospitalized earlier in the week for complications of a rare, painful autoimmune disorder and for atrial fibrillation, an erratic heartbeat that would spike dangerously. He was released from the hospital on Thursday with an appointment to return the following Monday morning to have his heart shocked back into rhythm, a procedure that had worked in the past when the heart rhythm medication had failed.

He had returned to work the following day, which was typical of him, and even made a day trip for a deposition. Clients were depending on him in nearly one hundred and fifty active cases in varying stages of litigation—mostly medical malpractice disputes in which he was retained by insurance companies to defend doctors and hospitals. He also headed and mentored a staff of younger lawyers.

Back at home that Saturday afternoon after lunch, while preparing for the party, Harvey tried sitting on a chair in front of a big blue cooler to nestle beer into ice. I heard him breathing heavily; he was unable to finish the job. He climbed the stairs to our bedroom and lay down on his back to rest.

As friends began arriving several hours later, I woke him to ask whether he felt like coming down to join us. From his sleeping position, he responded that he would be downstairs shortly. When he didn't show up within twenty minutes, I returned to check on him, but he appeared to have fallen back to sleep. Another twenty minutes went by, and once again I looked in on him. This time, he was awake, lying mostly on his back, with his right arm stretched out and flailing in the air. His left side was not moving. When I leaned over to speak to him, he mumbled through drooping lips what sounded like, "I can't get up."

I grabbed the phone to call Graham, a pediatric surgeon living close by. He and Lisa happened to be on a dinner date, and they arrived in less than ten minutes. Sprinting up the steps to the bedroom, Graham leaned over his father and asked gently, "Dad? Hey, Dad. How are you?" As Harvey tried to respond, Graham looked over at me and said, "Mom, call 911."

"What do I tell them?"

"Tell them your husband has had a stroke."

After calling, I could feel my blood pulsing and tried to breathe as I hurried downstairs. "Hey, y'all," I announced to our guests. "Harvey's not feeling well, so we've called the medics to take him to get checked out. You all just party on, and we'll keep you posted."

The neighbors began transferring food to the back of the house to give us privacy as an ambulance wailed to a stop in front of the house. Thanks to Lisa's calm suggestion, I packed a few things for Harvey, making sure to put his wallet with insurance cards and our cell phones into my purse. As the medics carted him out in his white tee shirt and plaid boxer shorts, seared into my memory is the sight of the neighbor who stood aside to close the door behind us. I never imagined that Harvey would not sleep in our bedroom again for 151 nights.

On the way to the hospital, I called our daughter, Ann, an attorney living three hours away in Raleigh. She threw some items into a bag and, with my sister, Jan, an attorney living in nearby Durham County, hit the road quickly. I don't remember how Graham was able to reach our younger son, David, a professor at the New Zealand School of Music, but David made immediate plans for the twenty-four-hour trip home.

By the time we arrived in the Emergency Department, the "miracle drug" called tPA was already dripping into his Harvey's veins to dissolve the blood clot that had formed in a lower chamber of his heart and worked its way into his brain. When we entered his cubicle, Harvey flashed a proud, crooked smile as he raised his left arm a few inches from the gurney.

"Wow. Look at you!" we said. "You're already getting better!"
How innocently optimistic we were.

> *April 14, 2013, 7:49 a.m.*
> *To: Family and friends*
> *From: Kandy*
> *Subject: Harvey*
>
> *I wanted to let you know that Harvey had a stroke last night. He is doing okay. He is in ICU at Carolinas Medical Center. Apparently, his atrial fibrillation, for which he was on medication, caused a clot to form which went to the brain. Fortunately, he got to the hospital in time (three-hour window) for a powerful clot-busting drug to begin working right away, and he improved right before our very eyes. He has some left-side weakness which we hope will improve over time....*
>
> *We will not be readily available by phone but will appreciate emails and especially your prayers. You know*

how private Harvey is, but I am taking it upon myself this time to communicate our news to the people we love and who love us. Ann is already here from Raleigh, Graham is with us, and David will be home from New Zealand Tuesday morning, and we will fight this together and "the old man," as they lovingly call him, will do his best, too. In spite of all he has dealt with, he continues to tell everyone in all sincerity that he is "the most blessed man on the planet." And a blessing he himself is! I will try to keep you posted with what I hope will be good news.

One of the first things we learned about strokes is that they can harm you in many ways. A stroke is the sudden death of brain cells caused by a blockage (blood clot) or a rupture (aneurysm, bleeding) in vessels that carry blood to the brain, depriving the brain of oxygen. The two sides of the brain control opposite sides of the body, so damage to the right side of the brain affects the left side of the body, right down the middle, and vice versa. Strokes on the left side of the brain can be even more devastating, because that hemisphere controls speech and reasoning.

Harvey sustained damage in the right middle cerebral artery. Fortunately, he retained his ability to speak and use his dominant right hand. He retained his long-term memory, basic reasoning ability, and personality with mild deficits. But it was as though his body were cut in half. He immediately lost the use of his left hand, arm, and leg. In fact, he lost all awareness of his left side: this is called "left side neglect." He no longer looked to his left unless reminded to. His ability to read was hampered, because he no longer automatically scanned to the far left of the page to find the next line of type. And, as can happen with any stroke, he lost his ability to swallow well enough to eat or drink without choking. Eventually—whether stroke-related or not—we discovered that he lost the vision in his left eye, as well.

There is a clear window of time—a matter of hours—in which tPA can start dissolving the clot and keep even more brain cells from dying. Then there is another window of time—optimally six to twelve months—in which the stroke patient must work to maximize recovery. Blood vessels and nerves can be trained to develop new pathways around the space that has been destroyed. At the end of the first year following a stroke, most of the possible recovery will have been accomplished.

Strokes can be mild, severe, even fatal, but many patients suffering strokes recover quite well over time. Had Harvey been dealing "only" with the effects of stroke, he probably would have progressed farther and faster in his recovery. Unfortunately, in the weeks and months that followed, his heart disease and other serious medical issues contributed to his disability and prevented him from participating in all the therapy he needed to regain what he had lost.

Complications

The workings of the human body are incredibly complicated, and its systems are intimately interconnected. A problem in one system can cause problems in other systems. But the practice of medicine is highly specialized, more fragmented than integrated. You start with a visit to your primary care doctor or, in a crisis, an emergency department, where a doctor orders tests and sends you to a specialist, who might order different tests and send you to another specialist. You quickly realize that many medical problems are difficult to diagnose and treat. Not uncommonly, Harvey's stroke was a broken thread in a web of medical problems.

In the beginning, an autoimmune disease that had taken years to diagnose responded only to steroids that damaged other parts of his body. Possibly caused by medication—possibly not—Harvey also developed atrial fibrillation. Possibly caused by the heart trouble—possibly not—he sometimes fainted upon standing, so falls became a big problem. Treatments and medications for different problems interfered with one another. And it all seemed to start with an afternoon in the sun...maybe.

After a bad sunburn on Hilton Head Island during a North Carolina Defense Attorneys' conference in 2005, Harvey began to experience periodic painful rashes, lesions, and large red bumps underneath the skin and in his joints, in flares that lasted weeks at a time. His hands and fingers would swell, or his lips or eyelids, or his throat. He would have trouble using his hands, especially for keyboarding. He ran low-grade fevers. He had difficulty swallowing. His face became mottled and puffy. He visited dermatologists, rheumatologists, and hematologist/oncologists. Blood tests confirmed inflammation in his system along with low counts of red cells, white cells, and platelets. He suffered what he called "exquisite tenderness" at sites of the swelling and significant pain. He received several blood transfusions.

After many tests and treatments over three years and several visits to Johns Hopkins Medical Center in Baltimore, Harvey was diagnosed with Sweet's Syndrome, a rare autoimmune disorder that affects mainly the largest organ in the body: the skin.

In the ensuing years, doctors prescribed almost every known medication for autoimmune diseases, from pills to infusions, from methotrexate to thalidomide, the latter for which he had to drive an hour and a half once a month to a major university medical center. We filled bulging file folders with insurance paperwork for the thousands of dollars some of these medications would cost. We fought through written and telephone conference appeals when prescriptions were denied. The medications arrived at our front door in packages of dry ice, or were dispensed in pill form at the pharmacy, or dripped into his veins at a clinic while he sat with his work on his lap.

But the flares kept coming, and the only medication that ever worked was prednisone, a steroid, in doses so high it damaged his body in other ways. Some days Harvey had to take four times the normally recommended dosage just to be able to swallow food or move his fingers. In the ensuing months, I found clumps of his hair in the shower; he developed the typical steroidal moon face; he had to be fitted for hearing aids; and ophthalmologists prescribed eye drops for glaucoma and performed surgery for retinal folds. Even though he took oral and intravenous medications to help reverse the side effects, the steroids thinned his bones and made him vulnerable to fractures, especially in his back.

One of the most dramatic side effects was the thinning of his skin. Just grabbing his arm could cause skin to peel off. Whenever he had blood drawn—which was often—the technician would cover the site of the needle with bandages and tape that stuck to the skin. When these were removed, the skin slid off and took weeks to grow back. Sometimes the wounds became infected. Wrapping wounds without tape or gauze of any kind is difficult and arduous. The only non-stick wound dressing recommended was very expensive, not available at most doctors' offices, and the insurance company accounted for it like gold coins.

Problems of the Heart

Harvey had an irregular heartbeat since childhood; I could hear it beating fast and then slowly, sometimes pausing, just by putting my ear to his chest. But it had not kept him from living a normal life. When he reached his mid-fifties, though, his heart rate became more erratic, and he was officially diagnosed with atrial fibrillation, an electrical abnormality of unknown origin. When the heart isn't beating regularly, blood doesn't flow smoothly through the chambers, and some blood can pool there. Pooling blood tends to clot, and a clot can then be pumped to other parts of the body, including the brain. In this way, a-fib is a leading cause of strokes. A-fib can be treated by medication or by shocking the heart back into rhythm. Over the years, Harvey's cardiologist tried both, but eventually neither option worked for long. He was not a candidate for a surgical procedure called ablation that can work for some patients.

To reduce the risk of clots and, therefore, strokes, in addition to medications to help the heart beat in proper rhythm, cardiologists generally recommend blood thinners for a-fib patients. When you take blood thinners, however—even small daily doses of aspirin—you risk significant bleeding in case of injury. For years, as a result of blood thinners, Harvey's right hand was purple-black from the pressure of handshakes that caused internal bleeding. Small cuts and bruises took weeks to heal. Meanwhile, the clotting factor in his blood had to be carefully monitored in countless trips to a clinic for blood draws. After each one, the medication dose had to be tweaked.

And then the fainting started. No one ever figured out why Harvey sometimes fainted upon standing. Countless tests of his blood pressure when he moved from sitting to standing were inconclusive. He never knew when it was going to happen. But at six-feet-four and two hundred forty pounds, when he fainted, he went down like a giant redwood. "If I start to fall, just move out of the way, honey," he would warn me, "because you'd be just a flea on the dog."

He had frightened more than one fellow attorney and client when he rose to his feet after a long meeting or deposition, took about ten steps, then passed out for several seconds. The first time I saw this, we had stopped on our way to the coast in pouring rain at a barbecue restaurant. After running from the car to open the restaurant door for us, I watched helplessly as Harvey walked partway to the entrance and then crumpled in the parking lot. I can still envision the hole in the wall of our study where his round head had crashed, and the blood that splattered on the walls and floors of our house from many falls to come.

Doctors would test diagnoses of "neurocardiogenic syncope" (heart-related) and "orthostatic hypotension" (blood-pressure-related), but none of the tests was definitive. So they struggled with a "catch-22" decision: do you give blood thinners to a man who is at risk for falling, thereby causing a fatal bleed in the brain or elsewhere, when he needs the blood thinners to keep his irregular heartbeat from causing a clot that could go to the brain and precipitate a stroke? To further complicate matters, because of the Sweet's, his platelet count was often dangerously low.

A few days before the stroke, during the hospital stay to deal with a severe flare of Sweet's, doctors discontinued Harvey's daily dose of aspirin as a blood thinner. The decision made sense at the time, but it turned out to be deadly. Since then, studies have shown increased incidence of stroke in a-fib patients in the days after blood thinners have been stopped. These complications ultimately caused him to lose his mobility, his career, his independence, and his life.

In the years leading up to the stroke, Harvey had told few colleagues and friends about his medical issues. But he didn't have to—they could see that he was not well, and we all worried about him. Even so, none of us predicted that the man we loved and depended on would work late one Friday night, have a stroke on Saturday, and never work again. That the next time he saw the mementos in his office, they would be packed in boxes to take home.

Deep and Sudden Changes

After the stroke, Harvey was, in many ways, still the guy we knew and loved. His ability to converse and remember remained largely intact. He continued to be witty, calm, kind, and comically opinionated. The clever one-liners never stopped coming. He rarely failed to thank every person who came into his room to help. For this, we will always be grateful. Yet he suffered irreparable damage to the "executive function" area of his brain, the part that affects upper-level thinking and reasoning, initiation, and motivation. He lost some of his ability to focus on details, multi-task, and navigate technology. He didn't seem as practical. He didn't seem to grasp the gravity of his situation. At times his personality seemed muted. Those of us who knew him well would say that he was just different somehow from that day forward.

Here was a larger-than-life person who had been in the shower before dawn six mornings a week for nearly forty years in order to be in his office by 6:30 a.m. Who had tried several hundred cases in courtrooms across the state. Who advised insurance company officials, medical professionals, and other lawyers; wrote briefs, spoke at hearings, and conferred with judges; flew across the country taking depositions, meeting with clients, and interviewing expert witnesses. Who counseled with hospitals and doctors to ensure that they performed and documented safe practices, according the official standards of care, for their patients. Who mentored many younger attorneys. Who helped anyone who called on him, day or night, for legal advice, and volunteered his time for those who could not afford basic legal services.

Here was a father who found time for his children's plays, concerts, ball games, and recitals. Who could converse in detail about classical and pop music, cars, sports, history, politics, medicine, and, of course, the law. Who drove happily to the North Carolina coast for boating, fishing, and walking on the beach whenever he could make the time.

Then, in a moment, he was draped in a gown, with wires and monitors dangling from all angles, machines beeping, his left side drooping, his long feet covered in too-small hospital socks and protruding from the end of the bed. Even though his career had taught him more about medicine than most lay people ever hope to know, he seemed unable to apply that knowledge to himself. Although he could hardly swallow and had nothing to eat or drink for days—and although he couldn't even sit up, much less walk—he kept asking to "go out for pancakes." Even though he remembered every detail of his cases, could still talk about composers and singers and sports teams and the people in his life, he kept asking us to bring his slacks and his car keys, to make reservations at his favorite restaurants, to rebook his work trip to Denver.

Over the next few days, his cognition improved somewhat, but his doomed optimism would stay with him for all the months he had yet to live. Was it hope, or was it brain damage? To the last day of his life, he was planning a fishing trip with a friend. He was going to renew his new driver's license and then buy a truck. Our family understood that some of his confusion was caused not only by the stroke but also by his difficulty in accepting his limitations. As days in the hospital ran to weeks with slow progress, we saw something else: the depression that so often comes with strokes and other serious illnesses.

Two other deterrents to recovery were his prior lack of physical conditioning and his size. With his health issues, heavy work schedule, and many years without regular exercise, he had not been in good shape before the stroke. Better muscle tone and strength would have enhanced his ability to work with the therapists toward improvement. Though not obese, he was a large person, difficult for aides and therapists to assist and move. It seemed they were always waiting for back-up. Even as he grew thinner in the months that followed, in each of the many medical facilities he visited or lived, whenever he needed to get out of bed, he was asked, "How TALL are you?" followed by, "I'll need to get more help." He had to be left in bed many times when he could have been encouraged to transfer to a chair or move around. We couldn't blame the aides for this; they had to be safe, for his sake and theirs. They had to follow the very rules their lawyer would have insisted they follow.

Another sudden hardship following major strokes can be difficulty with swallowing. We tend to take eating for granted. It's not just the food itself that makes meals important but also the habit of eating, the social contact it engenders and the way mealtimes order our days. So when we stop eating, a big part of everyday life is gone. Our family always enjoyed mealtimes together, with everyone participating in the preparation, snacking on chips with homemade salsa, putting together family recipes for meat loaf and potato salad, frying fish, grilling hamburgers or steaks, roasting fresh vegetables, and baking favorite desserts like cobblers, chocolate cake, soft cookies, and banana pudding. I typically cooked a hot meal for us in the evenings. Whether we were entertaining friends or merely eating on TV trays in front of a sporting event, Harvey rarely failed to tell me how much he enjoyed the meal.

The therapists determined that Harvey could not swallow safely after the stroke. Following nearly a week of intravenous feedings, with nothing by mouth, he was begging us to sneak in burritos and banana cream pie. He lost ten pounds in five days. But when the speech therapist offered tiny sips of water, even thickened, or the tips of spoons with tastes of applesauce and yogurt, Harvey choked. By the time his swallowing mechanism kicked in, the food or liquid was already sliding down the wrong way. He could aspirate and contract pneumonia.

> *Tuesday, April 16, 2013, 12:09 a.m.*
> *From: Kandy*
> *Subject: Re: Harvey*
>
> *Thank you to our wonderful friends for your words of encouragement and caring. I have read each message more than once. I'm sorry there isn't time to answer each one separately. It is incredibly busy here in the ICU, with doctors, therapists, nurses, and other staff in and out of the room all day long and into the night. None of us is getting much sleep right now, including Harvey.*
>
> *Many of you have asked for an update on Harvey's*

condition…There are several issues being addressed, including heart rhythm and weakness on the left side. The good news is that he still has all of his marbles! He is making jokes (he calls the neurologists "the stroke blokes") and aware of what is going on around him. The physical therapists ("animal trainers") got him sitting up today and even stood him up beside the bed. We hope to get out of ICU to a regular room sometime this week, and then to rehab to help him get his strength back. He is eager to get back home and back to work. It has been wonderful having Graham here to help with the medical issues. Ann took night duty the past two nights so that I could go home and get a few hours of sleep. We are all excited that David will land in Charlotte Tuesday morning. He happened to have next week off from teaching classes, so things worked out easily for him to come.

This is going to be a process, but we have lots of hope, and we are working on patience. You can't know how much it means to hear from you. For those of you who have asked, he is in Neurology ICU at (address), or you can send a card to the house (address). We think these will keep him cheered up a lot. The kids are already thinking up signs to post in his room.

Thanks to each one of you for your love and your prayers.

> Tuesday, April 16, 12:55 a.m.
> From: Kandy
> Subject: Re: Harvey
>
> One thing I forgot to say is that we can have NO VISITORS. ICU's strict rules. Only two immediate family at a time and we are already up to four (Graham fortunately counts as staff). We are dealing with serious issues including swallowing, speech, feeding tubes, managing heart and temperature, etc., constant visits by doctors and therapists, and many decisions. Harvey is very sleepy, also. But we love cards and all your kind messages. Thank you!

On the night of the stroke, a neurologist told us that the clot-busting drug was working. But he warned us not to be too excited about the immediate results, such as the raising of the left arm or wiggling of the left foot. Harvey's symptoms would get worse before they got better. The clot would eventually dissolve, and the bleeding in the brain would eventually stop, but swelling was occurring there, and a good bit of damage had already been done. The scans showed a large black area of the brain that had been destroyed—approximately thirty percent of the right side. Vessels would have to be stimulated to grow new pathways to circumvent the ruined part.

Ever the optimist, I thought that didn't sound so bad. Harvey was smiling (lopsidedly) and joking as always. He still had seventy percent of his right brain and one hundred percent of his left, and an excellent brain it was. His left arm and leg were moving a little. He was going to get well.

It was twenty months later that Graham finally told me of the bitter prognosis discussed with him by a consulting neurosurgeon late during that first night at the hospital: "Your dad might someday walk again; he might not always have to live in a nursing home."

Though we as a family normally don't believe in hiding the truth from one another, I was not upset that our son had not shared this. Because Harvey and I clung to the hope that he would improve, I encouraged him to work hard. Although it would have made the next two years and eight months easier for him in some ways, he might not have improved as much as he did, even for a short time.

What I do know is that, as hard it was, I was grateful for every day that he lived. There surely were days in which he wasn't glad to be alive, especially during the last months, but he never said so. He taught us about living authentically, gratefully, and graciously, no matter the circumstances.

Even Sick People Can Be Kind

> *Friday, April 19, 1:13 a.m.*
> *From: Kandy*
> *Subject: Update on Harvey*
>
> Since his stroke from a blood clot last Saturday, Harvey has remained in the neuroscience ICU. There are some tricky issues that the cardiologists and neurologists are dealing with. He remains in atrial fibrillation, which the

doctors believe is what caused the blood clot to originate in the heart. We hope there are no more clots, but he has not been able to have the TEE test for that because of risks. His heart rate is bouncing all over the place at a high rate, while his blood pressure is low. He can't be cardioverted into rhythm (which he's had twice in the past) because it could jar loose any remaining clots. He also can't start back on blood thinners yet because of the risk of increased bleeding at the site of the brain injury. We hope all of these issues will resolve very soon. There will be another CT of the head tomorrow and, if it's okay, he can be started on blood thinners through a feeding tube.

Our days are busy and we haven't had much rest. The occupational and physical therapists are helping him regain his strength in sitting up and moving some, despite the weakness on the left side, and he is doing well. Today he actually took a few tiny steps using the affected left leg. His left arm will need some work to get it moving again. He is talking a little bit better every day. They are working on getting him to move his head and direct his vision toward the weakened left side as well as the right.

His mind and his wit are still sharp. When one of the "animal trainers" held up a get-well card that said "Thinking of You" and asked him what it said, he replied with his eyes closed, "Get well soon." When she told him that wasn't right, he said, "Well, it ought to." She asked him again to try reading what the card said and he responded, "You're a sorry, sick old geezer."

He has already asked me to help him with a Guidebook for Stroke Patients. He says one section will be about what to do when you have a stroke. Examples:
- *Maintain a sense of humor.*
- *Let your medical staff and supporters know you appreciate them.*

And what to say to a stroke patient:
- *I care about you.*
- *I am praying for you.*

He has been an excellent patient until today, but he is really tired of being in the hospital. He has been asking for pancakes repeatedly. And he tries to trick us into helping him out of bed. We have had excellent care here—and this is not just because Harvey has represented them as an attorney for years!

Once he gets out of ICU, he will be in a regular room for a day or two before going into intensive rehab for a couple of weeks. We don't know how long his recuperation will take, but Harvey can hardly wait to get back home, back to the beach, and back to his work, which he loves. We hold these out as things to hope for and look forward to.

It will be awhile before he will have the time and energy to chat and visit. It has been wonderful having the kids here, and we keep each other cheerfully in stitches. Ann says we have probably shocked all the staff of the ICU with our irreverent jokes. But that's just us.

Harvey has a very strong faith, and we are praying

together as a family in his room each day. Please continue your prayers for comfort, healing, patience, and peace. We so much appreciate your words of love and encouragement. And thanks to each of you for caring.

"Shocked all the staff of the ICU" was an apt description of our family's behavior. In spite of the seriousness of Harvey's condition, our usual light-hearted banter and age-old family jokes kept our spirits up. There was actually an evening that a nurse came in to ask us to quiet down because there were people dying around us. When one of us later said, "I'm dying to go to that new restaurant," Harvey said, "Don't use that word jokingly around here!" Even so, you can read a lot between the lines of this latest emailed update. It's obvious that, by this time, we were all seeing just how bad the stroke really was and how difficult the recovery—to the extent there would be one—was going to be. You can sense the creeping fear that our life as we knew it was forever changed.

But the stroke did not take away the essence of Harvey. As usual, he was the center of calm in the storm around him. He was the person upon whom many of us had always depended in a crisis. His family and his legal staff relied on his judgment and steadfastness. His advice to colleagues during trials was, "Never let them see you sweat." Many times in the course of our long marriage he had asked me, a person prone to overreaction and hyperbole, "Why be calm when you can panic?" His conversation and comments were never impulsive, always judicious and thoughtful. He used to tease me, the spontaneous one, saying that I was like a gumball machine: "Every thought you have doesn't need to automatically fall from your brain and roll off your tongue."

It was not just his reputation at the hospital but also Harvey's uncomplaining attitude and freely expressed gratitude that made it a pleasure for his caregivers and family to help him. So often when I entered his room he would introduce me to the staffer there with something like "Honey, this is (name of person). She's been taking care of me all night. She has a cute little girl who is nine months old." He knew that patients can minister to caregivers, not just the other way around.

Harvey continued to deflect conversation from himself. Even when he was very ill, he asked his visitors, "How's your family? What do you hear from the kids? Have you done any fishing lately?" A few days after being hospitalized that first time, he asked me to look up a phone number so that he could call a friend on the anniversary of his daughter's death. Every person was equally important to him, from the couple who ran the dry cleaning business to the security guards in his high-rise office building to the trainee drawing his blood in the hospital and the doctor examining his eyes. I hope that, if I become ill and dependent, I will be as kind and grateful as he was.

While lying in one of many hospital beds, he began dictating to me more of what he wanted to write in his Guidebook for Stroke Patients. I still have the torn-out page from my notes that day. This is exactly what I recorded:

1. The importance of getting immediate medical attention.
2. The roles of various therapies.
3. How to relate to your family and friends. Let them visit

when appropriate; it's good for them and good for you. But not at first. When I hadn't made any improvements, I was just a sack of potatoes.
4. Remember to thank every caregiver, even if they're doing something uncomfortable to you. Being tossed around by the nurses up there—they have to haul you around in bed.

After a few days in ICU, Harvey was scheduled for a short procedure to have a feeding tube, called P.E.G., inserted just above the belly button to receive liquid nourishment and medications. On that day, another day of loss and disappointment, one encounter demonstrated that Harvey was still very much the smart, humble, ethical man we had always known him to be.

Ann and I had accompanied his gurney on the elevator ride to the surgical floor. As he was rolled down the hall, a nurse ran up beside him, calling out, "Mr. Harvey!" Surely he was barely recognizable to someone who had seen him only in suits and ties, upright, dignified, and in control. But he called her by name and was glad to see her.

"Is this your daddy?" she asked Ann. "This is my lawyer! He helped me so much. Always calmed me down and made me feel better. He is a wonderful man!"

Harvey was briefly put to sleep, the tube was poked into his belly, and we trooped back to his hospital room. Once he was settled, I commented, "That nurse sure did think of a lot of you. Did you defend her in a lawsuit?"

He replied, "I'm not at liberty to say."

As soon as the nurses began funneling the viscous yellowish

liquid from cans into the tube every few hours, Harvey's digestive system became upset. He continued to feel hungry and dreamed of eating real food. If an aide came to fill the tube when visitors were in the room, Harvey would say, "Pardon me for eating in front of you."

Even though he was the patient, I felt that he was handling the whole situation better than I was. A detailed person who likes to keep things orderly, I was frustrated that so much of what was happening was out of our control. I felt powerless and frightened. I wanted to be at the hospital with Harvey day and night, but I had to go home to sleep. I had to take care of the ongoing demands of our normal life in our household, as well as my own well-being. I began to see that managing our new, unwanted life—which we hoped would be temporary—was going to be an emotional and organizational challenge like no other we had ever faced.

CHAPTER 2

When a Loved One Becomes a Patient

> *Most people do not see things as they **are**; rather, they see things as **they** are...Most people confuse their life situation with their actual life, which is an underlying flow beneath the everyday life.*
> Richard Rohr, *Falling Upward*

Being Prepared: What I Wish I'd Known

When a loved one lands in a medical crisis, if you are the spouse or family caregiver, you are faced with many decisions during a time when you are least able, emotionally, to make them. Suddenly, you are a stranger in your own life. At the hospital or at home, you are attending to your loved one's needs around the clock. All sorts of people you never knew before are giving instructions you can't keep up with and asking for information you don't have, or don't remember. You lack the knowledge and experience to make all the decisions being required of you.

The patient might have to try different medications to see which ones work best, but side effects lead to even more medications and more specialists, so more names crowd onto your list. If you are at home, you can hardly keep up with prescriptions, how they interact and what time of day or night to take them, or with the people coming and going at all hours. Therapists with different specialties need to be scheduled to help with rehabilitation. You need to help the patient with everyday activities including walking, meals, bathing, and dressing. Your time is consumed with phone calls, juggling appointments, and ordering from the pharmacy.

Meanwhile, you worry about health insurance coverage, medical equipment, and changes to your home that might need to be made—for instance, providing wheelchair or walker accessibility with wider doorways, railings, and ramps; adjusting chairs and beds to optimal heights; remodeling bathrooms for handicapped access, and getting rid of rugs that can slip or catch under unsteady feet. You worry about money and transportation. You worry about your children, how they are coping and who is looking after their needs. Work at the office is piling up. Your car needs to be inspected, your grass mowed, your heating system checked, your gutters cleaned. Friends and family are calling constantly and they don't know how to help. The same people who have always needed you still need you.

And what about you? When do you eat and sleep? Should you spend the night in a chair at the hospital or should you go home? If you leave for a few hours, will you miss something important? You are feeling disoriented; your body feels stiff; you are exhausted. You crave fresh air. When did you last shower? Where did you park? Have the dogs been let out and fed? What's the name of that doctor who came by this morning? And where is your cell phone?

In those first days post-stroke, I didn't have any idea what I was doing. I was at the hospital most of the time, trying to figure out what was going on, communicate with everyone else who wanted to know what was going on, maintain a positive attitude, and basically "keep it together." I didn't want to believe that my husband was in a life-threatening situation, that he could be permanently disabled, so I just did not admit that possibility into my mind.

Managing all the details was a struggle and a challenge. I needed to keep up with Harvey's hearing aids, eyeglasses, CPAP machine for sleep apnea, both our cell phones and chargers, his various hospital room numbers, doctors, therapists, medical tests, clothing, communication with family and friends, two dogs at home, mail, and paying bills. I spent a lot of time tracking down and talking to hospital personnel about his needs while monitoring his therapy sessions, medications, and feedings.

I had to get organized. I began to realize how scattered our records were—some at home in various places, some at Harvey's office. He had routinely paid some bills while I had paid others. I needed names and numbers of his various doctors, insurance contact information, updated powers of attorney, online access to bank accounts, Harvey's computer passwords, and details of his disability coverage—only some of which I had at hand. In one day, I went from being vice president of the household to being president and CEO, and I wasn't ready.

Following is a list of things I wish we had done ahead of time to be prepared in case of medical emergency or loss of a spouse.

How to Be Ready for a Medical Emergency or Death in the Family

- Set up and maintain a family filing system for important documents, including legal, financial, medical, insurance, and tax records.
- Keep an up-to-date will, power of attorney, health care power of attorney, and living will for each adult. Store extra copies in your car's glove box or an accessible internet file at all times.
- Keep medical histories of family members, including dates of past surgeries, and store them in a safe place. Include names of providers and dates of service, test results, and medications.
- No matter your age, make notes about your wishes in case of death: funeral or memorial service preferences, burial or cremation, biographical information for obituary or announcement. Many churches and funeral services offer packets to guide you through this process and will store the information for you. This sounds maudlin, but planning removes stress at a terribly difficult time.
- Keep a secure record of all internet passwords for yourself and your spouse. Know how he or she paid bills and learn how to access online banking. When possible, put

accounts into joint names with "right of survivorship" provisions.
- Keep family tax records in one safe place and learn about your financial situation. Discuss how you will manage financially if one of you becomes ill or disabled. The partner who usually prepares the taxes needs to share the details with the one who does not.
- If possible, establish a relationship with a financial advisor who can keep all this information for you and knowledgeably help with the important financial decisions you will have to make. You don't have to be wealthy to do this. If you haven't already, consider a relationship with a CPA who can furnish information on what records to keep for tax purposes and the dates tax payments are due throughout the year, as well as prepare your tax returns for you. The percentage retained by financial and tax advisors is well worth the fees, especially when you are overwhelmed with the day-to-day responsibility of caregiving.
- Learn all you can about your insurance coverage, including disability. According to what you can afford, develop a plan for contingencies, including acute and chronic medical conditions, prolonged hospitalization, and disability.
- Purchase pill organizers and use them. Pick one day of the week to set up medications for the week. And be sure to make required changes that might be prescribed by doctors in the meantime.
- Establish a relationship with a pharmacist you like and trust.

- Keep on hand a supply of thank-you cards and stamps. If you are blessed with many caring friends, you will want to use them. Also purchase a supply of get-well and sympathy cards or, better yet, a supply of blank notes to write on. You will come to realize just how much these expressions of love mean during hard times, and you will make the time to send them.

Communicating with Family and Friends

One of the first things we have to decide when illness strikes is how best to communicate with family and friends. Whom do we need to contact? Whom do we want to tell, and what do they need to know? We want to include family members, neighbors, co-workers, close friends, and people whose names are on the calendar of the sick person and immediate family—people who are counting on us for activities and commitments we can no longer carry out, at least for a while. We must decide which persons to contact for help while we are dealing with the crisis—those who will assist us with work and volunteer responsibilities, children, pets, lawns, trash day.

Normally, I spent enough time talking to my friends on the telephone that the kids dubbed me "Mouth One" and a close friend "Mouth Two." Since I have what Harvey called "a voice that carries," he used to suggest, "Why don't you just hang up and stick your head out the window?" However, in a medical crisis, I knew that I couldn't personally phone every person who needed an update, even if I wanted to. We needed a system. Or, as my daughter would quote my well-worn mom-mantra, "We need to get organized."

On the morning after the stroke, I telephoned a few family members and colleagues, then sent the first of what turned out to be a series of **group emails**. Being able to get the word out to many people at once was a great convenience. Harvey and I discussed the advantages of letting people know what was happening. Though he had been such a private person, he surprised me by agreeing to the emails because they would meet three important goals.

1. Group emails let friends and family know what is happening in exactly the way we want them to know, which lessens speculation and second-guessing and controls the flow of information. Remember that old childhood game of "Gossip"? It's best to get your message straight in order to minimize misinformation. That way, even private people can formulate statements they are comfortable sharing.
2. The emails help avoid too many phone conversations. We eliminated countless hours of retelling the story and answering questions.
3. For those who want to help, the group messages communicate the needs and wishes of the patient and the family.

A pleasant consequence was that a number of our friends began to respond by email. I enjoyed sharing these responses with

Harvey and the children. Those who received my emails began forwarding the messages to others who might be interested, and people began asking me to add them to the list. My technology skills and my time were limited, and I probably never used the same list twice. So some **help setting up a list-serve or website link for updates** would have been nice, and I've added that to my list of helpful things to do for sick people and their caregivers.

I didn't use **CaringBridge**, because I thought that was for people with serious long-term illnesses—which, of course, wasn't going to be our situation at all. But CaringBridge and similar websites are excellent ways to keep communication going. I began to use Facebook as well, but my messages there were understandably not as personal or detailed as the emails sent to our selected group of recipients.

Meanwhile, our daughter began posting updates on Facebook. She found that, with the appropriate privacy controls, Facebook could be a good way to keep people updated on her dad's situation. I include some of her posts in this book as they advance the story while revealing, with poignancy and humor, the feelings and perspective of an adult child supporting her parents during some very difficult times.

April 20, 2013
Ann's Facebook Post

For those of you who do not know: My sweet dad had a stroke on April 13 and has been in ICUs since that time. We are so fortunate that he is one hundred percent the same guy we know and adore. In typical Harvey and

Kandy Cosper fashion, Mom and Dad have been unwavering in their strength and steadiness and are handling this situation with the utmost grace and humor. Dad has made marked improvements, especially in the past few days, and we're hoping he'll be out of the ICU, into a regular hospital room, and into rehab very soon (perhaps as soon as the end of the week!). If you feel moved to help, we can have NO VISITORS and do not need any food at this time, BUT cards, emails, and prayers go a long way, as well as flowers, balloons, etc. When Dad comes home from rehab, our needs could change in terms of help, food, and visitors. We can't answer all of your messages right now, but please know that they mean more to us than you will ever know and we cherish each one. Please message me if you would like Mom and Dad's address, email addresses, etc. It's going to be a long road, but we are ecstatic about his improvement and very hopeful about his recovery. Keep sending up prayers for the big guy—my hero, my mentor, my rock, and just generally the best dad ever.

Practical Suggestions for Caregiving Family Members

Among the most important items to keep with you at all times, in addition to a **cell phone and charger**, are **small notebooks with pouches** in which to record names of doctors and therapists and their instructions, lists of people who called or visited, items you need from home, items you need at the pharmacy or grocery store, reminders, appointments, funny or poignant comments from the patient, and anything else you will want to remember. The pouches can hold business cards of medical personnel, chaplain, social worker, pastors, wheelchair salesmen, and a host of others who come into your life.

Today I still have six or seven small notebooks from those days filled with names, dates, and numbers. They contain scribbled lists of people who called, sent flowers or food, or brought gifts, with check marks affixed when I thanked them. These notebooks are vital for caregivers, because there is just too much happening at once, too much to remember and comprehend. As soon as the doctor leaves the room, you forget her name and you forget what she said. You can't remember who the occupational therapist was or what days he said he'd be coming. Or who dropped by for a visit, or who you were supposed to call to make a follow-up appointment, or what the patient asked you to bring from home, or who at the insurance company asked you to call back.

If you are going to be spending time in medical facilities, purchase a **washable lightweight bag to take with you everywhere**, knowing it will be on your shoulder, or in the back of a car, on the floor of a bathroom or hospital room, underneath a chair, behind a bench outdoors, hanging from a walker or an IV pole. When it slides across the floor of the emergency room or gets splattered with Diet Pepsi (or worse), it can easily be washed.

In addition to holding your notebook, phone and charger, the bag also can be stocked with some re-sealable sandwich bags (for everything from hearing aids and reading glasses to cafeteria leftovers), ballpoint pens, rubber bands, paper clips, protein bars, little prayer books, medical forms, tissues, blank thank-you notes and stamps, lists of medical providers and their contact information, address stickers to identify personal items, informational handouts, copies of medical forms, a water bottle, slipper socks, a paperback book, and the all-important notebook. If you take a Kindle or iPad, be sure to attach your name and address sticker to it and other belongings in case you become separated from them. Thanks to a friend who brought them to me, I practically lived with one of these bags hanging from my shoulder.

Another recommendation, when patients are going to be in the hospital for longer than a day or two, is **personalizing their rooms**. From a doctor's perspective, Graham advised us that **photos and cards help medical staffers to see patients in the context of their everyday lives.** Bringing in family pictures and displaying get-well cards are ways to help the staff see the patient for who he or she is. Ann made funny posters, the grandchildren drew pictures, and we propped up a few family photos wherever Harvey was "incarcerated," as he called it, at the time. He loved directing attention to them, and they communicated to the staff that he was a beloved husband, dad, granddad, colleague, and friend. Across the painted cinder-block walls of his room, we strung hundreds of get-well cards he had received. Sometimes Harvey was too sick and depressed to notice them, but I enjoyed them. I know that these glimpses into his personal life meant a lot to him, to the people who assisted him, and to the family. The mementos also gave the staff a starting point for questions and happy conversations about family and friends. One friend whose baby granddaughter was hospitalized for a long time purchased materials so that her family could spend some of the long, tedious hours creating colorful origami birds that they strung across the room.

When it became obvious that the hospital stay and recovery process would last a lot longer than we had expected, I set three rules for my own survival: **eat some kind of meal with protein three times a day, go home to sleep every night, and exercise for a few minutes every day**, even if that meant walking hospital halls, leaving my car at the back of the parking deck, and taking the stairs between floors. As long as I followed those three rules, I had the energy to do what was needed for Harvey. I have friends who make different choices, even sleeping on the floor at the hospital, especially when the sick loved one is a child. That wasn't best for me during this time. It's important for us to feel free to make our own decisions.

The hospital cafeteria offered a wide array of good, fresh choices for meals and snacks, but the times I could get down there varied according to what was going on with Harvey. I rarely took food into his room, since seeing and smelling "real food" is a mild form of torture for hungry people not allowed anything by mouth. When possible, I slipped across the street from the hospital to walk along the greenway for a few minutes of exercise and fresh air, but this did not happen every day. Occasionally, friends would put themselves on call to pick me up on short notice in front of the hospital and take me out for a quick lunch or supper close by.

Tuesday, April 23, 2013
From: Kandy
Subject: Re: Update on Harvey

There is a children's story that Graham reminded us of today. A woman goes to the wise man complaining that her teapot whistles. The wise man tells her to go home and get a goat. She comes back to complain that the goat screams and the teapot whistles. So he tells her to get a cow, but the cow moos, then a horse, etc. You can see where this is leading. Eventually he tells her to get rid of all the animals. She is delighted to report how quiet her house is with the lovely, soft whistle of the teapot.

This is the perspective we have today—a day of good news and thanksgiving for the Cosper family. You might not know that, over the weekend, Harvey was moved from neuro ICU to cardiac ICU, because his heart rate was high and wildly irregular. It is this a-fib that caused the stroke in the first place and could have caused another one at any moment. Today the doctors were finally able to safely perform a procedure to look at the heart and check for more clots. Since there were none, they were able to shock his heart back into rhythm. If it stays in rhythm, he will be moved to a regular room tomorrow and on to Carolinas Rehab next door by the weekend. He needs inpatient rehab to help strengthen his weakened left side and get him sitting up, walking, and talking better in order to resume his good life.

Humor continues to abound. When the nurse told

Harvey that, if he would work hard at sitting up, he could rest all afternoon, he responded, "I don't negotiate with terrorists." Ann told Harvey that, with all his wires and plugs, he looks like the back of her TV right now. Then Harvey, who was trying to stand up with the IV pole and wires, said he was "line dancing." When he awoke from the heart procedure today and learned it had worked, he snapped the fingers of his good right hand and sang, "I've Got Rhythm."

Right now we don't need anything except your continued prayers and encouragement. God has spoken to us especially through each of you. We love hearing from you. No visitors yet, please. We will let you know when he changes rooms again. THANK YOU for your love and caring. That and God's grace will continue to sustain us on the road to recovery that stretches ahead of us.

Somehow, now, the fact of recovering from a stroke seems like a whistling teapot.

Learning To Be an Advocate

As astute as Harvey was about the field of medicine, he was not well enough to keep up with all that was involved in his care. **It's important for every patient to have an advocate—a parent, spouse, other family member, or close friend who knows him or her well and can assist in communication between the patient and the medical staff.** Someone who functions as a second set of eyes and ears to help interpret what the professionals say and remember details of the diagnosis, prognosis, treatment options, patient responsibility, and requirements. Someone who will record doctors' explanations and instructions, help the patient understand the purpose of medications and treatments, and communicate any special needs the patient might fail to mention.

In our case, we were fortunate to have a surgeon in the family who was constantly monitoring his father's situation and communicating with medical colleagues. He slipped in and out in his green or blue scrubs between operations, sometimes in the middle of the night, more often than I will ever know. Always with his light-hearted, down-to-earth attitude, he helped in every possible way. But as the wife, I assumed the role of daily caregiver. I appointed myself Harvey's official round-the clock advocate and supporter-in-chief.

I lacked some characteristics of an ideal caregiver, including patience, calm demeanor, gentle nature, and ability to respond with equanimity to the unexpected. But I possessed three qualities that were important: a high energy level, tenacity, and loyalty to my husband; at least two of Harvey's caregivers described me as "feisty." I did not always endear myself to the professionals who looked after him, but I insisted on explanations and results. I wanted to understand every medication and procedure ordered for him. I wanted to know the people treating him, what they were doing, and why. I wanted his every need met. When we rang the call bell, I expected a reasonable response. When therapists were scheduled to work with him, I expected them to come on time and help him make progress. But I quickly learned just how difficult the job of advocate was going to be for me. I had to recognize that, in facilities full of sick people, we were not the center of the medical universe.

Hospitals are mind-numbingly busy places. People are in and out of patient rooms at all hours of the day and night. Patients are rolled from floor to floor for tests and procedures as they pass food carts, lab technicians, doctors in scrubs, cleaning crews with linens piled high, clusters of families laughing and crying, nurses sharing notes, portable computer terminals, machines being wheeled in and out of doorways and elevators, even children running around and yelling. There is little difference between day and night as phones are ringing, people are talking in the halls, and—most persistent of all—IVs and monitors are constantly beeping. Staff members call to one another in the long hallways and engage in full-voice discussions outside patient doors at all hours. Sleeping is difficult for the exhausted patients. Pushing the call button does not guarantee that a busy nurse or hard-working aide will be available for simply routine care anytime soon, whether it's to stop a beeping IV or get the patient to the bathroom.

I spent some time each day **keeping up with the personal items and organizing the clutter** of the small rooms, moving stacks of clean towels and gowns from the sink or the only extra chair to the closet; tossing syringe caps and latex gloves that had fallen to the floor; removing pitchers of ice water that still came even for a man not allowed to drink anything; finding nooks in his bedside tray table for his reading glasses, hearing aids, phone, lotions, patient information booklets, and a toothbrush no one else remembered to help him use; locating electrical outlets for his CPAP, and positioning flowers sent from friends.

Hospital pharmacies were unable to mix the special eye drops he needed to treat the glaucoma and retinal problems, so, in every place he stayed, we had to get permission to bring in the eye drops, leave them with the nurses, then remember to take them with us when he was moved or discharged. I tried **monitoring prescribed medications**—which ones he was taking and why, who had prescribed them, what side effects to watch out for, and how they interacted. This was very helpful later on, when I had to dispense them to him at home. And, although it was uncomfortable at first, I learned to help him with the urinal.

It was rare to be treated by the same nurses and CNAs (Certified Nursing Assistants) several days in a row, especially when the staff worked three twelve-hour shifts per week, instead of five eight-hour shifts. Harvey was moved many times within hospitals, and everyone was always very busy. So it was often difficult to establish a rapport, and I became accustomed to saying "he needs a bed extender to keep his feet from hanging off the end" and "let's post a sign to remind everyone he can't have tape on his skin." But when it was possible, **getting to know the hospital staff and medical team** was a blessing to us. Harvey remembered better that I did the names of those who helped him, and he made sure to introduce them. They appreciated his kindness, gratitude, patience, and humor. Some of them did not appreciate the meddling wife, but I felt that I was doing my job.

I learned about the following people who, in addition to

the team of physicians, would be crucial to the well-being and improvement of my stroke patient:
- nurses
- certified nursing assistants (CNAs)
- physical therapists (for gross motor skills such as walking and transferring, flexibility, and overall strength)
- occupational therapists (for fine motor skills and activities of daily living such as dressing and bathing)
- speech therapists (for talking, swallowing and cognition/reasoning)
- social workers (for all patients and their families)
- respiratory therapists (making sure breathing is safe and oxygen or CPAP machines are properly hooked up when needed)
- imaging specialists
- phlebotomists (blood draws)
- housekeepers
- food servers
- and hundreds more behind the scenes, dispensing medications, keeping records, receiving visitors, preparing food, and performing countless other tasks on the patients' behalf

In all the facilities in which Harvey was treated over a period of nearly three years, we had mostly positive experiences with competent and caring staff. These professionals have many people to care for—not only patients, but distraught families, as well—and they do an excellent job meeting so many needs. In spite of long hours, hard work, challenging patients and family members, and unpredictable interruptions, they go home after their shifts to their own living situations with their own needs, problems, families, and responsibilities. Most are to be lauded for their dedication and willingness to take on such challenging, life-affirming jobs.

Sometimes, of course, errors and oversights do occur; and the more closely the advocate is following the patient's care without being intrusive, the more likely that human mistakes can be caught and corrected. Almost every day, for instance, someone managed to put tape on Harvey's fragile skin—and, when removed, that tape pulled off the skin. Many times, calls for assistance stretched out so long they became emergencies. I spent a lot of time in the hallways seeking out help and asking questions.

Several months after the stroke, a new nurse in one facility failed to give Harvey the proper evening medications. Within six hours, his resting heart rate spiked from 64 to 148. When I returned the following morning to find Harvey breathless and agitated, I had his heart rate checked and, immediately upon reading the results, the staff called an ambulance to rush him to the emergency department. When I asked to see his chart, I discovered that the CNA who checked the heart rate the night before had merely recorded the alarming numbers on a sheet of paper and left it in his medical file. The nursing supervisor definitely heard from me about that. Another time, Harvey had a nighttime caregiver to whom he referred as "the Big Nasty" because, he said, she was gruff and physically rough with him. He could not, or would not, give me her name, and I wasn't there at night to confirm this. But I did discuss the situation with the nursing supervisor, who found it to be true and took appropriate action.

Though these incidents were rare exceptions, they demonstrate why an advocate's job is especially important to the safety of the patient. The majority of the time, we felt blessed with excellent care from trained professionals who dedicated their lives to helping others. We admired and enjoyed getting to know them.

Keeping the Peace

As Harvey's advocate during those long, hard days, I tried to **remain upbeat, hopeful, and calm**. Not for the purpose of putting up a front, but to keep up Harvey's spirits, along with my own and those of our children and close friends. Normally extroverted, busy, and talkative, I had to learn how to sit quietly and companionably for hours—a **presence not requiring anything** from him. Harvey had never been a chatty person, and peaceful surroundings were important for him. "Too much talking" agitated him even more after the stroke than before. Some years earlier, when Harvey was asked at my brother's rehearsal dinner what advice he would give to the bride who was joining the family, Harvey said, "The family did not know I had vocal cords for the first three years of our marriage. If you ever want to get a word in edgewise, I would advise you to master the fine art of interruption."

An example of this dynamic had occurred one afternoon

several years before the stroke when Harvey told Ann and me with great pride that he had repaired a ceiling fan in our den. He began to describe in mind-numbing detail the flywheel in the fan and the intricacies of getting it to work. Bored after the first sentence, Ann and I kept rolling our eyes toward each other as his explanation went on and on. Harvey finally looked up and said, "What?" We burst out laughing. Then he said, "Everyone else in this family talks all the time. But let me put more than two sentences together and everybody's complaining that I'm talking too much." From that point on, whenever Harvey or anyone else started to explain anything in great detail, we called it a "flywheel story."

Harvey was never fond of constant flurries of activity, no more so than when he wasn't feeling well. He had often said over the years, when my frantic activity around the house interfered with his relaxation, "Why don't you alight someplace? You keep jumping around like a flea on a hot brick." During the many long weeks in institutions, I began **reading aloud** to him. I made sure to leave the room to use my cell phone when I knew that conversation would disturb him. I took walks in the hallways.

I was keenly aware that this new part of our life together was about Harvey—his medical problems, loss and pain; his work toward recovery, his desire to get back to work, and all the complications that were standing in the way—and, most of the time, I did not resent it. Although my life had changed overnight, mine was the easy job. Mustering all his energy to get through each day with new disabilities while doing the hard work required to get better—his was the unfathomably difficult job. To my distress, it began to appear that Harvey might not be up to tackling it.

Had I been the one to suffer a stroke, I believe I would have awakened every morning with one goal in mind: work hard to get better. However, Harvey was exhausted and depressed. The "motivation center" of his brain was damaged. So while I was pushing him and everyone around him to help him recover, he wanted to rest. This dynamic was frustrating for both of us. But my role as advocate required me to **be encouraging without pushing too hard**.

Another important job of the advocate is to **help control the flow of visitors**. I was uncomfortable telling family members and friends that Harvey didn't want to see them at first. The few who came, anyway, were apologetic once they saw his difficult situation. We appreciated those who responded with understanding and without taking it personally. But after we allowed visitors, we were grateful for the diversion, the fresh air from the outside world, their smiling faces, new and interesting conversations. I learned to **move towards the door and say, after about ten or fifteen minutes, "Thank you so much for taking time to come by. It was so good to see you."**

Though I had complained about the time and effort required in **filling out forms** and chasing down busy doctors to complete and sign them, the disability insurer confirmed that, since Harvey was unable to perform normal "activities of daily living" or ADLs (I started throwing around terms like this with the best of them) such as dressing himself, he qualified for expanded catastrophic benefits. I would be able to cover the cost of home care and required renovations with these funds.

Finally, the advocate must also begin to **make plans to assure that home will be safe for the patient who eventually will be able to return home.**

The Importance of the Immediate Family

Keeping the best parts of the family dynamic intact, if possible, reassures the sick person that life will go on for the family in a spirit of love, even in the toughest of times. It establishes a foundation of support and encouragement for one another.

In addition to the spouse or main caregiver, members of the immediate family can help immensely just by being present—in person, by phone, and via the internet. Adult children can find their own unique ways to contribute while continuing, as best they can, with the demands of their everyday lives. In our case, the cast of characters for this role was our three children.

Graham, a busy surgeon, was frequently on call day and night, and a husband with small children, but somehow he found time to slip into his dad's hospital room at random hours whenever Harvey was in the hospital. Harvey never failed to tell me when Graham had visited him if I had not been present. In his green scrubs and cap for one hospital, or his blue outfit for the other one, Graham offered a cheerful, relaxed presence, a sense of humor, a deep faith, and a medical knowledge that reassured us. He was always deferential to the medical staff and to us in making decisions about care. He never tried to take over or tell other people what to do. But we knew Graham was quietly consulting with the staff to closely follow his father's situation. He lovingly checked over his dad, performing small tasks to make him more comfortable. His prayers at Harvey's bedside encouraged us and reminded us that God was with us always.

Having David home from across the world cheered us immensely. His quiet, loving presence, sensitivity, and humor helped to keep us optimistic. He always seemed to know the right thing to say and the right time to say it. He and his dad shared a great love of music, listening to it and talking about it, and an interest in history. Hearing about his interesting life in a beautiful country on the other side of the world—a place we had visited him—fascinated us. Soon he would have to return to teaching in Wellington. How very difficult it must have been for him to leave. Although the rest of us had to carry on in the hard reality of the day-to-day experience with his dad, we at least were present. After he flew back across the International Date Line, the seventeen-hour time difference would make it difficult to find convenient times to call, but he made it work, and every Skype visit and phone call lifted our spirits.

Ann, an attorney for a state nonprofit in Raleigh, drove the three hours to Charlotte every weekend for months. The sparkling personality of his "baby girl" charmed her father and never failed to cheer us and our helpers, even in the darkest of times. Throughout the week, she called her dad at least once a day to offer encouragement and love, and she spoke to me separately at least once a day, as well. She could always engage him in "lawyer talk" that kept his mind stimulated even if they were like "flywheel stories" for the rest of us. She sent cheerful, encouraging messages and made funny posters for his walls. Sometimes she would slip into my bed when we got home from the hospital exhausted late at night, and we would talk, laughing or crying, or just breathe side by side. She was a practical help always; but, even more, she spread sunshine whenever she came. She also posted updates on Facebook that gave our friends a fuller view of what was going on with us.

Like their father, our children share a relaxed, commonsense approach to life that always manages to find the humor in a situation. I worried about them, the emotional impact of seeing their father so ill and helpless. I worried about the disruption in their busy lives and careers. I knew they worried about me, too. It was harder to "be there" for them as their mother when I was struggling with fear and grief myself. But their steady support and encouragement helped keep me grounded, and they enhanced not only the quality of their father's life but, I have no doubt, the length of his life, as well. Whenever we were together, we always found things to laugh about.

April 23, 2013
Email from Ann to Mom
You are an incredible wife, mother, human being, and servant of the Lord. I can only hope that someday I have half of the love, energy, fortitude, and sparkle that you bring to every aspect of your life and to the lives of others. You are a true steel magnolia; you are my hero, inspiration, and friend. You can do this. See you tomorrow.

April 23, 2013
Ann's Facebook Post

Sometimes life is so hard you can barely breathe. And you can't be grateful, and you can't be hopeful, and you're not sure life will ever be the same. And it may not be. But the resiliency of the human spirit is undeniable, irrepressible, and unexpected in its depth, and love and compassion can take over in ways you never knew you or others were capable of. It's the emotional equivalent of the average citizen having the strength to lift a car during an emergency.

There's a lot of pain in the world, but I personally am constantly reminded that I am blessed beyond measure with a lot of things, namely the best family in the world, the gift of laughter, and the ability to delight in small successes that indicate greater things to come. Sometimes, you have to live on prayers and hope, even if you're not sure anyone's listening. But you take a deep breath and wake up the next day. And the next day. And the next. I have peace in knowing that God is good, and that is my prayer for the world right now.

Chapter 3

When a Friend Becomes Ill

In this life we cannot always do great things. But we can do small things with great love.

Mother Teresa

First Responses

When we first hear that someone we care about is ill, facing a medical crisis or a diagnosis of serious illness—whether in the hospital or at home—our first inclination might be to contact the family or even the patient. Letting them know they are loved and thought about is important, of course. We want to know what's happening, we want them to know we care, and we want to help somehow. For the patient and immediate family, knowing others care is vitally important. However, dealing with the medical, physical, practical, and emotional impact of serious illness is stressful and exhausting. Responding to constant calls and texts, repeating details over and over, telling what happened and what the doctors are saying, can add pressure. So families appreciate it when loving friends **minimize phone calls**. Cards, emails, and text messages can be preferable to calls, especially when they do not require a response: **"Please don't feel you have to return this message; I just wanted you to know I'm here for you."**

It's important for the patient and family to be able to control what is said and what is known about the patient's condition, treatment, and prognosis. Not everyone needs to know the details of a patient's symptoms and condition. Extrapolations by friends and acquaintances are not helpful. So families appreciate it when their friends **respect the patient's privacy by repeating only what is said by the patient's family,** rather than passing along guesses, opinions, or conjecturing to others. A welcome note might say, **"I care about you and want to help in whatever way I can. Let me know if I can help communicate any information you are comfortable sharing with others and any needs you might have."** With patients' permission, we can **add their names to prayer lists and let other friends know they are unwell without going into painstaking detail about their illness.**

Visiting Sick Friends

Whether in the hospital or at home, sick people might not be getting much rest. Even for members of the extended family, it's thoughtful to **ascertain whether visits are encouraged. If they are, they can be scheduled for short, convenient times. Even for members of the extended family, if the patient or family asks for no visitors, we provide them with kindness**

by honoring their wishes. Many find it exhausting just trying to talk, much more so to entertain guests. Not only that, but circumstances requiring privacy come up throughout the day at unforeseen times. The hospitalized patient might be resting, using a bedpan, having a catheter checked or a dressing changed. The patient might be engaged in an important conversation with a doctor, therapist, caregiver, minister, parent, child, or spouse.

Those of us who want to visit are providing them with kindness when we accept their wishes without being personally offended. **"Crowd control" is important for people who are hospitalized.** I have seen many patients' rooms so crowded that families spilled out into the hallways, blocking traffic, talking loudly, with children crying and running in the hallways. They stayed for hours, often well into the night, and disturbed the patients in nearby rooms. In our case, Harvey needed rest in the times that staff was not attending to him, and he wanted privacy. For him, this was not a time for noise, long visits, and chatty conversations.

When Harvey did not want to see visitors, I was tempted at first to push him with a guilt-inducing "But they insist on seeing you and I promise they won't stay long." But I respected his wishes, even when I had to be the bad guy. It was difficult, when people had made the effort to come and braved the mind-boggling parking lot, to leave them standing in the hall. So it was helpful for people to **check with the family ahead of time** to see whether they should come—close colleagues from the office, for example, who could reassure him that his clients were being well cared for.

If the patient is not ready for company, friends can send a card or an email. Simple messages of cheer and encouragement are appreciated. Suggestions about what to say and what not to say are included in this chapter and the one that follows. Today, several years later, I still have all the cards that people sent over his thirty-two months of illness. I had always planned to re-read them with Harvey. I still hope to do so, and now I am doing it alone.

When visitors are welcome, they go a long way in stimulating patients and their families, bringing fresh air from the world outside and lessening boredom. If the patient asks for short visits, this means less than ten minutes. In the hospital, there probably won't be a place to sit, anyway. If there is room for another chair in the room besides the battered non-functioning recliner reserved for the spouse, it's going to be covered with stacks of linens, plastic syringe bags, and pieces of tubing. One long-time friend used to come to the door and just stand quietly in the hall for a few minutes. We could see him there, his concerned look, his kind smile, his hand inching up in a little wave. And then he would be gone. Fred's presence was a powerful expression of love, though he rarely even came into the room.

Don't bring anything to the patient in the hospital unless it's requested, especially not food. Patients not in intensive care might enjoy balloons or flowers or gift baskets, when permitted, but there is so little space in the room. Inpatient hospital meals are not generally known for their gourmet qualities; it's impossible to serve fresh food at optimal temperatures to hundreds of people three times a day. But the meals are planned to meet the required dietary needs of the patients.

The only exception to this was when people checked with us beforehand to see whether they could bring something for family members to eat. In those cases, our friends either left food in a cooler on our porch at home or brought it to the hospital for us at pre-arranged times. But we were always careful not to eat in front of Harvey during the weeks that he was denied food. The hospital cafeteria offered healthy, tasty, reasonably priced foods, and it provided the family with a change of scenery for a few minutes when we were able to get there.

If patients ask for visitors, please come! So many people wanted to visit in those first weeks of hospitalization, when it was best not to come. But when we did ask for visitors, later on, it was wonderful to see them. The conversation stimulated Harvey, bringing him news of the outside world and much-needed rapport with people other than family and medical personnel. In his quiet way, Harvey never failed to entertain his visitors as much as they entertained him.

Harvey: "Have you been doing much work lately?"

Semi-retired attorney friend: "I worked a couple of hours on Monday."

Harvey: "You're running circles around me."

One of the few people we invited to visit during the first weeks after the stroke was a younger attorney with whom Harvey had worked closely for almost fifteen years. They had sat together at many a courtroom defense table. Harvey could not rest until he had spoken with the other members of the "med mal" team about all the work that had to be done on behalf of clients—Harvey's active cases in addition to the ones that the rest of them were handling. They reassured him that the clients would continue to be well-served. They told him that opposing counsel were thoughtfully allowing postponements in cases coming up for trial. I could hardly imagine the extra hours those men and women were putting in to keep things proceeding smoothly at the office. Although they wanted to spare him from worrying, Harvey never tired of getting their updates, and he seemed to remember every small detail of every case.

It was difficult for these colleagues to see their mentor weak and disabled. But their reassurance was one of the greatest gifts Harvey received throughout his illness. They helped him feel that he still had something to contribute, even while he had lost so much. After some of them left Harvey's room, we stood outside in the hall together and cried.

What not to do

> *Many of us 'helper' types are as much or more concerned with being seen as good helpers than we are with serving the soul-deep needs of the person who needs help. Witnessing and companioning take time and patience, which we often lack—especially when we're in the presence of suffering so painful we can barely stand to be there, as if we were in danger of catching a contagious disease. We want to apply our 'fix,' then cut and run, figuring we've done the best we can to 'save' the other person.*
>
> Parker Palmer,
> On Being, "The Gifts of Presence, The Perils of Advice," blog,
> April 27, 2016

When a Friend Becomes Ill

The most important thing to realize about people who are ill is that we cannot "fix" them or their situations. Unless we are their doctors, nurses, or therapists, it's not our job. Though I am speaking here about situations of illness, this is true for other situations of suffering, as well. As family members and friends of people who are sick, we want to make the situation better, but often we don't know how. As a result, we sometimes say and do things that are unhelpful and, occasionally, even harmful. Insisting on doing something they don't need or want is satisfying our own needs, not theirs.

I wish I had understood this years ago. I cringe to think of all the things I've said to suffering people in trying to make them feel better, because I couldn't stand to see them hurting; in truth, I was trying to gloss over the unpleasantness and make myself feel better, as well. The times I've talked about myself, my family, people I knew, when all they needed me to do was allow them to do the talking—to listen. The times I've tried to force them to "look at the bright side" when all they needed was a hug. The times I've truly cared about people, thought about them, and prayed for them, but never let them know—never stopped them at church to tell them so, never called or sent a card, or dropped off a container of soup. I just hope all those people for whom I made awkward gestures of caring, or whom I failed to acknowledge at the time, understood how hard it is to leave our own comfort zones and enter another's pain. That so often we mean well, but we just didn't know what to do.

Before describing all the wonderful things people said to us and did for us—a story that would fill a whole book in itself—I feel it's important to mention some rules I learned which could be called "what not to do."

As I was doing informal research for this book, surveying and talking to people who had been through hard times, I always asked, "What is the number one thing people said that you didn't want to hear?" Following are guidelines based on what I heard most often. The first one is the most important but least followed rule for being a friend to others in their time of need.

1. **It's best to resist the temptation to make the conversation about ourselves or other people. We honor hurting persons by staying present with them in their situations.**

One sunny spring day not long after Harvey's stroke, I escaped from the hospital long enough to take our dogs for a walk. A passing neighbor stopped in her car and rolled down the window.

Neighbor: "How's Harvey?"

Me: "He's hanging in there. Today the therapists were working on getting him walking again."

Neighbor: "We have a friend about his age who had a stroke five years ago, and he still can't walk."

After a moment of shocked silence, I couldn't stop myself from responding, "That's not helpful."

It reminded me of a comment made to my mother once in a cardiologist's waiting room. A fellow patient asked, "What is the reason you're here?" When Mom replied, "I have cardiomyopathy," the woman said, "Oh, my cat died of that."

When a Friend Becomes Ill

A week or two after my mother died some years later, I ran into a friend who told me she was sorry to hear about my mom. Then, she cried as she talked about her own mother's health problems. After listening for a long time, raw and in the depths of grief, I finally excused myself. She said, "We'll get together soon and talk more about you." But we never did. Her mother lived for years after that.

I don't know why so many of us do this. As soon as we hear about a problem, we mention someone else who experienced it. We exclaim, "Me, too!" Or "My friend has that." We start talking about some ailment we've had, or our grandfather's sister-in-law's cousin. You can't find a Facebook post about a person's problem without reading comments in which others respond about themselves.

I believe many of us do this because we truly are trying to establish a connection: we think this shows that we understand. But what we might not realize is that responses like this can be ways of closing the door on the suffering person. Perhaps their struggle is too hard for us to face, and it's certainly easier to talk about ourselves. As discussed in Why I Wrote This Book and Our Life Before, our stories do build connection. But there is a later time for us to share personal stories. Suffering people first need to be acknowledged, listened to, and affirmed in the uniqueness of their own situations. They are having enough trouble handling their problems without having to respond to other people's pain, too. People receiving bad news and people having a hard time need most of all to know that others care about them.

In other words, when we hear about the trouble of another person, the first thing out of our mouths should not be about what happened to us, our aunts, our dogs, or our spouses. This can make people feel like small fish in a big pond of similarly suffering people. When they are one-upped with "anything that's happened to you has happened to me, only worse," this minimizes their problems. Unfortunately, running off on personal tangents displays a lack of empathy, as though we are able to see life only from our own limited experience and viewpoint. This is particularly unhelpful, and sometimes hurtful, for suffering friends.

Once I saw this happening to Harvey and me, I became acutely conscious of how often we—and I'm including myself here—immediately switch the focus of conversations to ourselves, making ourselves the heroes of the story, eager to share something similar, or better, or worse. When I started paying attention to this, it became like hearing a dripping faucet: I couldn't stop noticing how often people engage in parallel conversation instead of reflecting and responding to each other. I began to see the value of the applying the WAIT theory: asking myself "Why Am I Talking?" Suggestions for active listening are included in the next chapter.

2. **"I know how you feel" is not usually helpful.**

Almost every person I surveyed mentioned this: don't tell me that you know how I feel. No two people and no two situations are exactly alike. Again, instead of forming a bond, presuming to know how another person feels can be interpreted as "there's nothing special about your situation; you're just one of many." For me, I already knew that millions of people have had strokes. But this was my husband, my family, my deep pain. Hearing about other people's strokes just made it worse.

Of course, some of our circumstances are similar, and sharing information and feelings can be comforting. A general comment such as "It's unbelievably hard seeing your spouse suffer" shares some understanding without making it all about us. We share empathy in comments such as "Your life seems so different now, doesn't it?" and "It is so hard for all of you in your family to have to go through this." Perhaps we can make reference to a remarkable coincidence: "I learned about strokes in caring for my husband, too," or "Long hospitalizations can be so stressful." But our own storytelling will be more welcome later, in more relaxed circumstances. Later, we can ask permission to share similar stories—when they have time, when they are emotionally ready to do so.

3. **It's best to avoid asking personal questions, seeking details.**

A number of people I interviewed expressed surprise at the personal questions they were asked during times of illness, especially by people they barely knew, from acquaintances to casual friends to customer service employees. Sharing details about illnesses and other life experiences might be common on talk shows and in celebrity magazines these days, but such private information is ours to share only when we are comfortable doing so. It puts people on the spot to be asked for information that others really don't need to know, and it can come across as mere curiosity instead of true caring. Best to express our concern and allow the patient or family member to share as they feel comfortable.

4. We need to be careful about giving unsolicited advice.

Most of us want to be helpful to others. But when we begin making suggestions and giving unsolicited advice, we are implying that we know their situations better than they do, better than their doctors do, and are better prepared to make decisions about them than they are. Although it might make the giver of advice feel helpful and important, it can make the receiver feel defensive. Expounding on what we or other people have experienced, what we've read on the internet, which doctors are the best, or which herbal remedies to try is not going to fix them. They already have plenty of experts telling them what to do. As frustrating as it is, we must accept that there are other ways to help suffering people we care about.

Jumping in with advice when we first hear of a friend's diagnosis makes it about us, not them. We are talking, not listening. Every situation is different and people have their own medical teams, their own issues, their own needs. What we have to share might be more than they need to know at the moment, overwhelming, discouraging, going against their own doctors' advice, or just plain irrelevant. Giving them our lists of possible diagnoses and cures is inappropriate. We can let them know we are willing to share information or similar experiences—if and when they are ready.

After Harvey became ill, I was amazed at how many lay people suddenly became medical experts. I might be working my way around the exercise machines at Curves, responding to well-meaning questions about how Harvey was doing, when someone who had never been to medical school, never had a stroke, never even met Harvey might proffer some glib advice such as, "You just need to get him a walker." I wanted to answer, "Wow! Why did none of the fifty-three medical professionals helping him ever figure that out?" Depending on how grouchy or overwhelmed I was feeling at the moment, I might have pointed out, "Well, since his left arm and hand are paralyzed, he can't exactly hold onto a walker."

Eventually, I worked out a better way to respond: "We have excellent providers who are doing all they can to meet his particular needs right now." What this implies is, "We understand that you want to help, but this is not the best way. We don't need you to suggest that we go to different doctors, try alternative healing methods, take more vitamins, or call an elderly friend of yours who had a similar experience nineteen years ago in South Dakota."

People questioned why I didn't get more help at home, or move Harvey someplace else, or fly him out of town for a second opinion, or try out any of numerous other remedies and ideas. But, unless they specifically ask for advice, what sick people and their caregivers appreciate from their friends is affirmation and respect for their need to make their own decisions about what is right for them.

Sometimes we try to mask the fact that we are giving advice by phrasing it as a question: "Have you thought about..." or "Have you tried...." Again, this puts the patient and family on the defensive, requiring them to give more personal information or explain why the suggested action was or was not followed. And many people are uncomfortable sharing those details. When others offered me advice, I did not want to sound ungrateful by responding that we had faith in our ability to make decisions based on the professionals' recommendations; that their ideas were not helpful, or that we had already considered them and cast them aside. But sometimes I wanted to put up my palms in a "pushing away" motion that begged, "Please stop."

In a blog entitled "The Gift of Presence, The Perils of Advice," well-known writer Parker Palmer said this:

(1) Don't give advice, unless someone insists. Instead, be fully present, listen deeply, and ask the kind of questions that give the other a chance to express more of his or her own truth, whatever it may be. (2) If you find yourself receiving unwanted advice from someone close to you, smile and ask politely if you can pay a little less this month.

Of course, those of us who have gone through similar experiences often have helpful suggestions. Sharing our stories can be bonding and loving. With the permission of the patient or family member, these conversations can take place in more optimal times and places, after the original crisis, when the shock has subsided and the prognosis is clearer. Ideas on the best ways to offer helpful suggestions are included in Chapter 4, "Ways to Show We Care."

Unwelcome Platitudes and Comments

When people we know are going through hard times, we often just don't know what to say. So we find ourselves coming up with platitudes that aren't helpful at all. We must not beat ourselves up if we remember having made these statements to other people but, going forward, we can be more sensitive to what we are implying. Not everyone going through hard times will agree with my list below, but I have found very few people who find comfort in these statements.

- **Anything starting with "At least…."** When we try to force a suffering person to "look on the bright side," we minimize the physical and emotional pain they are experiencing: "At least he's alive…at least you have good insurance… at least you're not in a lot of pain…" The other person could be thinking, "But I didn't want to be sick in the first place!"
- **"Everything happens for a reason."** I realize this might be comforting to some people, but it's not for many others. What would be the reason for a child to die of cancer? For a tornado to destroy a town? For a hard-working family to become homeless? For a husband to have a stroke? Is it someone's fault, or God's fault?
- **"God doesn't give you more than you can handle."** This

also might seem comforting to some people, but not for many others. It suggests that God caused the suffering in the first place. Harvey and I never blamed God for illness and suffering. People going through hard times are wondering how they can just get through another minute of the day. It can make them feel guilty, resentful, or angry to believe that a supposedly loving supreme being would deliberately test them by inflicting pain. Contrary to popular belief, this exact saying is not in the Bible. What Romans 8:28 says is this: "We know that all things work together for good for those who love God, who are led according to his purpose."

- **"We don't understand why God causes these things to happen."** I do not believe that God deliberately inflicts pain on us. If I did, I would be very angry with God and tempted not to believe in him anymore. Psalm 34:18 assures us that "the Lord is close to the broken-hearted and saves those who are crushed in spirit."
- **"You must be feeling (exhausted, discouraged, angry)."** It's best not to guess at or ascribe feelings others might have; we might actually make them feel worse. Instead, we can be open to their telling us how they are feeling.
- **"Let me know if there's anything I can do."** People in crisis may not even know what they need and, if they do, they are not likely to feel comfortable asking—especially not picking up the phone at a later date and calling someone. They may not even remember who offered. In our case, my first two attempts to ask for help were embarrassing. The first time

was obviously an inconvenience to the helpers, and the second time several people turned me down; they all had good reasons, but it had been difficult enough to ask for the help, and I was discouraged from trying again.
- **"Call me after the procedure." "Let me know how things are going."** For me, I was so busy and distracted that I was lucky if I could keep even the immediate family in the loop.
- **"I haven't heard from you."** This statement feels accusatory. I hope no one took my lack of communication personally. Often I didn't even remember whether I'd taken a shower that day.
- **"What are you going to do about...?"** People in the midst of a medical crisis are trying to just get through the day. It's best not to question them about the future. Questions about future plans ("Are you going to stay in your house?" "Will Harvey try to go back to work?") were hard for us to answer.
- **"You've got this! You're going to beat it. You can do it."** Several dear friends struggling with cancer have told me recently that this kind of cheerleading, while certainly well meant, can be heard as false, unhelpful, and guilt-inducing. Sometimes called "dismissive positivity," these statements do not fool people whose serious and even life-threatening health conditions are not within their control to heal.
- **"You need to take care of yourself. If you don't, you won't be any good to anybody."** This is well-meaning advice for the advocate (parent, child, spouse, or other caregiver). For

Harvey, he was doing the best he could. For me, I knew my limitations and made a decent effort to take care of myself. I also figured out what was best for my family as we worked through it all, day by day. But for a time I had to put Harvey's immediate needs ahead of everything else. And I'm glad I did.

- **Inappropriate humor.** We make all kinds of jokes in our family, about almost everything; we have few sacred cows. We are generally light-hearted. But the middle of a crisis is a touchy time to try humor that involves the patient and family. Example: "Harvey sure went to great lengths to avoid buying you a birthday present this year."
- **"Did you get my card?"** Busy, stressed people in crisis are dealing with many details and human interactions every day. They appreciate every gesture and expression of caring, but they don't always remember who sent what.

Many, if not most, of us have in the past said some of these things to people going through hard times. We must forgive ourselves and hope those to whom we directed those platitudes have forgiven and forgotten. Until we go through hard times ourselves, we don't truly understand, so we just do the best we know how. Suffering people are grateful for the support, kindness, and love of others, even when awkwardly expressed. They probably don't even remember what we said; they just remember that we cared. But, going forward, there are more meaningful ways to express concern and show compassion.

Engaging With Faith

Before you speak to me about your religion, first show it to me in how you treat other people; before you tell me how much you love your God, show me in how much you love all His children; before you preach to me of your passion for your faith, teach me about it through your compassion for your neighbors. In the end, I'm not as interested in what you have to tell or sell as in how you choose to live and give.

U.S. Senator Cory Booker,
Facebook Post, April 24, 2012

It is important not to romanticize a person's fear and painful experience by speaking in spiritual terms that can leave the person who is hurting feeling unseen and unmet. At a very basic level, any real response to suffering must always include letting the hurting person know sincerely, 'I am so sorry you are having to go through this painful experience...'.

Fr. Richard Rohr, Center for Action and Contemplation,
"Daily Meditation, October 25, 2018," adapted from James
Finley, Thomas Merton's Path to the Palace of Nowhere

Of course, sometimes when bad things happen it is a consequence of our own actions. But we should be very cautious in attributing our suffering to God, or in believing that suffering is God's punishment....Just as you would not inject cancer cells into your children to teach them or punish them, neither does God give us cancer....God does not send suffering our way, but

> *God can use it and work through it. As we invite God to use our suffering, and to bring good from it, our suffering takes on meaning. We find strength to bear it and sometimes even joy in the midst of it.*
>
> Adam Hamilton, *John: The Gospel of Light and Life*

If we mention religion to people who are suffering, it's important to make sure they share our beliefs. You will notice that several suggestions of what not to say have to do with God. People's understanding and perception of God varies greatly. We all know folks of different faiths and folks of no particular faith. Since our own beliefs may not be the same as those we are trying to comfort, our religious statements can disturb and alienate suffering people at a time when they are most vulnerable. Some people find great comfort in their faith during hard times, while others find their faith challenged. Hard times tempt many people to doubt their faith, to wonder where God has been, and to chafe at the mystery of why bad things happen to good people. We honor those who are suffering by respecting their personal beliefs without trying to convince them of ours.

As a Christian, I believe that God welcomes our prayers and that prayer can change things, especially inside those who are praying. I am grateful for the gift of life and its many blessings, and for God's guiding, loving presence with us in all situations, both good and bad, when we are open to him.

I am always surprised, though, when people thank God for things that are good for them and terrible for others: "God saved our home in the hurricane," "God saved me in the accident," "God cured my child's cancer." But where was God for the people whose homes were destroyed, who died in the crash, or whose bodies were ravaged by disease? Why didn't God save them? For us, we never believed that God sent the blood clot to Harvey's brain, any more than we believe God kills families in car wrecks, or inflicts children with cancer, or sends tsunamis to destroy cities; any more than we believe he wills certain sports teams to win or people in a hurry to find parking spaces near the grocery store.

Many people I love and respect, including other Christians, believe differently. Some are convinced that everything that happens to us, including every bad thing, is part of God's plan. They find this comforting in accepting illness, suffering, and death. For us, we accept the biblical prophet's words that our thoughts are not God's thoughts, nor are our ways God's ways. God's workings are a mystery to us. It's enough to know that God is present with us at all times and his love works within us through all circumstances. God strengthened Harvey and kept him in his everlasting arms. Harvey and I felt God with us every step of the way, and that knowledge was comforting. The prayers that we said privately, with each other, and within the family, with our ministers and with friends throughout the day, were full of gratitude and not so full of requests.

Instead of engaging in theological discussions, we can offer simply the ministry of presence. We can take our discussion cues from those whom we wish to comfort. Most importantly, if we are praying people, **we can let our friends know when we are praying for them.** For Harvey and me, this was the best thing people could say. Some people also told us that God was with us. But, honestly, we already knew that.

April 30, 2013
From: Kandy
Subject: Re: Update on Harvey

  The week since my last update has been filled with ups and downs, and the long days and nights have run together in our memory. A day or two after his cardioversion into sinus rhythm—eleven days after his stroke—he was cleared to leave ICU for a regular room. In the ten minutes it took to roll his bed through the halls and transport him by elevator from the seventh floor to the sixth, his heart lapsed back into atrial fibrillation at a high rate. We knew immediately, because the nurse for his room on the new floor ran an EKG strip, then rushed out of the room to call the doctors. It took several more days of balancing medications to get the heart rate back down, the clotting factor safe, the blood pressure high enough, and so on. Although the staff continued limited occupational, physical, speech, and swallowing therapy, as each long day in bed ticked by, we were concerned about losing ground in recovery.

  Yesterday was a banner day. By late afternoon, Harvey and two nurses and I made the trip through the tunnel from the main hospital to the rehabilitation building next door. He is in a big, sunny room in a spotless, well-run facility. For at least two weeks, he will be put through a rigorous boot camp of various therapies for strength and mobility: sitting up, standing up, walking, using his left arm and hand, talking (already pretty good), and swallowing. He is fed and administered medications through a P.E.G. in his stomach; he has lost twenty pounds, and he is dreaming about all his favorite foods and the restaurants he will enjoy when he can get out and eat again.

The plan is to reassess in two weeks and perhaps even come home then. They will let us know what we will need to do at home to be ready for his long-awaited return. Perhaps we should have added a downstairs bedroom to our older home instead of the kitchen and porch renovation we just finished last year. But we will work things out when the time comes.

When I asked Harvey what to tell you in this latest update, he gave the "thumbs up" sign and said, "Tell them I am still fogging the glass." And thank God for that! He continues to crack everyone up with one-liners, including the animal trainers. In all these seventeen days, he has not once failed to thank a single person who has come in to help, whether it be to clean his room, draw blood, give medical updates, or a thousand uncomfortable maneuvers and procedures he has had to endure. I am proud of his spirit, his character, and his determination, and proud to be his wife.

As for the family, about which so many of you have been kind enough to ask… the staff has commented more than once on the family dynamic, and we are blessed with *these children and their love.*

The doctors, nurses, technicians, all the people here have been professional, caring, and accommodating. And not just because Harvey has helped them out a good bit over the years! Even the cafeteria food is good - and believe me, I am an expert on it now. The fourteen-hour days in the hospital have come to an end, and I am so happy about that! Although it's been fun to see each new nurse or assistant come in, gasp, and ask Harvey "How tall are you?" before calling for backup. And did you know that there are bed extenders available in the hospital, but it's nearly impossible to get XL rubberized socks?

Believe me when I say how much your love and caring mean to us. We love cards and messages. Since rehab is exhausting, visitors are limited. If you want to visit, please email me and we will try to work out a time. Otherwise, we continue to cherish every expression of concern. The long days are strung together with the signs of God's love through our family, friends, medical staff, ministers, and each other.

Harvey sums up the experience so far in this way: "Every time someone has come in to ask me my name, birthday, where I am, and why I am here, I have gotten the answers right. And I am grateful for that." Yesterday he told me had dreamed, again, that he was cooking sausage and eggs in the kitchen for our breakfast. These are small dreams and goals for a big person. We decided that we would never again take for granted those small things that go on in an ordinary day—things we surely will be able to do again one day.

You enjoy those small things in your day today. And God bless each one of you.

Chapter 4

Ways to Say We Care

The human soul doesn't want to be advised or fixed or saved. It simply wants to be witnessed—to be seen, heard and companioned exactly as it is. When we make that kind of deep bow to the soul of a suffering person, our respect reinforces the soul's healing resources, the only resources that can help the sufferer make it through.

Parker Palmer,
On Being, "The Gifts of Presence, The Perils of Advice," blog,
April 27, 2016

The Gift of Listening

Years ago, during a group training exercise at a nonprofit for which I worked, our leader gave the participants a topic to discuss. There were two rules: no one could interrupt and, before speaking, each person had to summarize what the previous speaker had said. After one person started off the discussion, the next person had to begin with, "What I heard you saying was…."

This exercise was more difficult than you might expect, because we actually had to listen to the previous speaker; we couldn't simply be thinking of what we were going to say next. My family would surely tell you that I didn't seem to learn a whole lot from that exercise, but I actually did—it's just harder for some of us talkers to follow those rules. In most circumstances—especially when we are speaking with someone who's going through a hard time—this reflective listening is an important gift.

When we are truly listening, we reflect feelings based on what the other person has said. We enter that person's story. The best way to connect with others is not so much to share our own experiences as to show interest and caring in their unique situations. For example:

Friend: How are you feeling?
Patient: I'm doing better, but I feel so tired.
Friend: It's probably hard for you to get much rest.
Patient: I have some pain, and people are in and out of the room all the time.
Friend: Oh, I'm sorry to hear that. It must be really tough. I expect you have good doctors and nurses who are helping you with your pain and your recovery.
Patient: Yes, they are really good here. Therapy is hard work.
Friend: You have several therapists?
Patient: Oh, yes. They get me out of bed and exercising every day in all sorts of ways.
Friend: Isn't is funny how things that make us better can be such hard work? But I have great faith in you.

Patient: Thanks. I hope you're right.
Friend: I hate that you are having to go through this. So many people are thinking about you and rooting for you. I bring you love from all the people who miss you at (office, neighborhood, church group, or wherever).
Patient: How is everything going there?
Friend: (brief news from the outside world) Well, you get back to resting up. It's so good to see you. I'll be back in touch soon.

The proliferation of support groups attests to the benefits of sharing—not advice, but experiences and feelings. There is a time and place for this. But, **in conversations with struggling people, the best thing to do is listen. We can bestow compassion, a gift from the heart.**

If they don't want to talk further about themselves and their challenges, then they will redirect the conversation by asking us questions or bringing up another subject, as Harvey always did. Our willingness to go elsewhere in conversation with them is another gift we can give. We can then offer them a glimpse of the outside world beyond their own confining situations.

It's best not to presume how others feel or what will make them feel better. When a friend is in a tough place, instead of barging in, we can wait to be invited. We can offer the gift of presence—not just once, but consistently over time.

A young woman I know was recently diagnosed with breast cancer. I understood and appreciated her Facebook post announcing the news in a way that protected her from an onslaught of personal comments. Anticipating that most respondents would immediately mention the experience they or other people had with cancer, she clearly stated that she did not want any advice, suggestions, or personal stories; she just wanted us to know.

Two years after Harvey died, I lost my beloved little dachshund, Mister Hankie, who had provided us with seventeen years of humorous antics, love, fun, pee stains, walks, and sneaking under our covers every night. Stories about Hank were legendary among our friends, and I wanted to let them he was gone. But I dreaded that telling them would precipitate a flood of sad personal stories about their own lost pets. So I ended my Facebook post with this: "It would be very hard for me to read responses to this post about the pets you have lost in the past, because right now I am already too full of sadness. But I am sorry for all of us who have lost our best furry friends, and I know how grateful we are to have had them in our lives."

Of course, we can learn much from each other. There is practical information from which patients and family certainly can benefit. For example, "We found reading aloud to be a good way to pass the time," or "There is a little coffee shop at the other end of the hospital that has really good quiche on Fridays." Or "our church offers free handicapped equipment. Just keep it in mind in case you need anything."

From personal experience, I know a good deal about medical and rehab facilities in our area—what they are really like and how they compare. I can suggest practical things a caregiver can do to stay organized once an illness hits in order to make life a little easier. So I have learned to say, **"If you think you might be** interested, just let me know and, when it's a better time, I'll be happy to share what was helpful to us."

When a friend's husband suffered a serious stroke not long ago, I passed along a couple of practical suggestions that I thought would be helpful. But she has never sought me out since. It turns out that her situation was different and, in some ways, more devastating than mine. I am still learning the difficult lesson that we cannot be surprised or offended when people do not want our advice. We can become sensitive to their signals: their eyes will glaze over, they'll look away and sigh, they'll make excuses to end the conversation, or, in written communication, they will not respond.

For me, though I rarely sought or welcomed advice, I was comforted by the presence of people who cared, people who talked about my husband with affection and love, people who decided on little acts of kindness they were comfortable doing and then just did them. Most of all, I will never forget the friends who just stood with me and cried.

Expressing Concern

Following the stroke, I was asked hundreds of times: "How's Harvey?" Everywhere I went, from church to supermarket, and almost every time I answered the telephone, I heard, "How's Harvey?" I was so grateful that people cared about us, and I understood that people wanted to know how things were going. I wanted others to care about him. I was consumed with his situation; it was my life, as well, and it was good to talk about it at times.

But I found myself repeating the same news over and over again. If I tried a short answer like "he's hanging in there" or "we hope he'll be home soon," the inquirer usually asked more questions, probing for more details. It was difficult enough to live through this hard time without having to talk about it so much.

Illness can take over your life. You so much want—yearn, even need—to be the same person you always were in your former everyday life. You don't want to give up your identity. You want to have normal conversations and experiences. You want to be reassured that the everyday world is still there, and you are still a part of it. And yet, you do want people to understand that you're having a hard time. I realized there was a way to let people know you care without demanding anything from them or putting them on the spot.

Instead of asking a question, we can make a statement: "I have been thinking about you." That way, they're not required to give personal details if it's uncomfortable to do so, but it leaves the door open for them to say more if they choose to. For me, I enjoyed normal conversations that let me know the real world was continuing on pace, even while I was living in caves of caregiving for months on end. And Harvey always preferred to hear about other people's lives than to be grilled about his own circumstances.

I do not mean to suggest that we should ignore the other person's struggles and pretend they haven't happened. I found it awkward when I ran into acquaintances who chatted cheerfully about other subjects without a mention of our circumstances, as though nothing out of the ordinary had happened. Then I felt obligated to mention Harvey's condition just to make sure they knew. To the good old Southern "How are you?" I would answer, "It's been tough since my husband has been sick." It's important to acknowledge the problem, to name the elephant in the room. But after concern is expressed, moving on to other subjects is good. As time went on, I added many people to the group emails that updated folks about Harvey's condition, and this helped a lot.

I have friends who report that, when they were caregivers for sick family members, many people asked about the sick person but not about them. **It's important to recognize the pain and challenges of those who are caring for sick loved ones, but not in an advisory or judgmental way.** I became uncomfortable when people came up to me with intense expressions on their faces and asked, "How are YOU doing?" Usually I gave an abbreviated "Oh, I'm hanging in there all right." What was I supposed to answer? How do you think I'm doing? Fine? Not. Do I really look that bad? The real answer was, "My husband had a stroke and it has wrecked our life." Their question was often followed by, "If you don't look after yourself, you won't be any good to him."

I appreciated their acknowledging that my life was, in many ways, as challenged by Harvey's illnesses as his was. I was doing what felt right for me, and that was enough. I rarely responded with the full truth: "I'm discouraged, sad, exhausted, longing for some free time without worry, overwhelmed with details, scared to death, and just trying to hold it together one day, one hour at a time." No one wants to hear all that. Once again, a statement was more appropriate than a question. Better for the caring friend not to ask how I was doing, but to say, **"It must be so tough on you, too, and I pray for better days for you both."**

Some people would say, "I'm inspired by your energy and devotion," or "you are so strong." These are kind, encouraging comments, and I appreciated that other people recognized my devotion to my husband. But at times those comments evoked guilt. I knew that I was no hero. Sometimes I was feeling resentful, impatient, and discourteous. I had dark, depressed moments when I felt neither energetic nor devoted, and certainly not strong or inspiring. I was doing it all out of love, yes. I was doing the best I knew how. But I also didn't have a choice. I had to get up every day and do what needed to be done, even when I choked back tears throughout the day, grieving at seeing my strong husband so weak and helpless. Even when I wished for just one day, one hour, to myself. I needed people to recognize that what I did was sacrificial, yes, but that I was flawed and human—and love me, anyway.

We especially appreciated **messages and gestures of concern that do not require a response**. I could thank friends for their concern by text or email at convenient times without being interrupted during a feeding, doctor visit, therapy session, or much-needed rest. I read aloud to Harvey all the responses to our group emails, and all the cards we received, and we felt blanketed by love. Here are some comments that are always good to hear.

- "I'm awfully sorry you've got this going on, and I'm one of a lot of people who are pulling for you." (Harvey's favorite)

- "I love you."
- "I am here for you."
- "I hate that you are having to go through this. You have many people who care about you."
- "I have been praying for you." "We pray aloud for you every night at dinner." (if you actually do)
- "I know you have a great medical team."
- "I'm sure you're making the best possible decisions for your situation."
- "It must be so hard for you right now."
- "I think about you so much."
- "I'm so sorry. I wish I could make it all better for you."

But what we say is less important than how we listen and what we do.

Practical Help During Serious Illness

Although there is little we can do inside the hospital or sickroom to foster healing, there are outside chores that can be very helpful. **We can perform the mundane, everyday chores of life so the patient and family can focus on the medical situation.** Because the families of seriously ill people are stressed and busy, when we are offering to help it's a good idea to make it clear that we understand if the patient or family doesn't have time to respond: "I'm here for you. If I don't hear back, that's okay; I'll be in touch later on."

Rather than ask what they need, it's a good idea to think of something we would like to do and then just do it. From my experience, following are examples of what to say that include practical ways to help:

- "I can pick you up in front of the hospital for a quick lunch out tomorrow. Text or call me when you think it's a good time for you to slip out."
- "I will drop off your favorite sandwich or salad. Just see how your day goes and text me when it's a good time."
- "If I can run errands for you on Friday, please send me a list."
- "I'm on my way to the store. Let me know what you need."
- "If it would be helpful, give me a list of people to call for you."
- "I will text you on Monday morning to see what I can do for you that day."
- "I don't cook, but name me your favorite restaurant food and I'll bring it over tomorrow."
- "I left a small bag on your porch for you" (baked goods, wine, journal, an apple, a little book of devotions, peanut butter crackers, note cards).
- "It's a gorgeous day for a walk to the park. I can be in Harvey's room any time this afternoon if you want me to sit with him while you get some fresh air."
- "I'm available to walk your dogs any afternoon this week."
- "I rolled out your trash cans for pickup tomorrow."
- "I watered the ferns on your porch."
- "I have extra flowers I'd love to plant for you."

Ways to Say We Care

How blessed we were! Friends thought of so many ways to add smiles to our long days. One close friend hand-delivered a card to the house every day for the first couple of months. Another sent a card every few weeks for more than two years. Remarkably, a dear couple sent a vase of colorful flowers at the beginning of every new hospitalization or rehab—at least a dozen cheerful arrangements arrived from them over the next thirty months. It got to the point that, as soon as our friend identified herself on the phone to the florist, the owner would immediately ask, "So where is he now?"

Many people offered practical help to make the days easier. One friend left a supply of cooked bacon and hard-boiled eggs every week for a while so that I could quickly fortify myself with protein in the morning before zipping out to the hospital. Neighbors planted colorful flowers around our mailbox and patio so that when I came home the house looked cheerful. One of Harvey's co-workers drove to our house after work one day with a bucket of supplies to wash Harvey's pollen-covered car, one swipe at a time. Another friend dropped off cinnamon bread fresh from the bakery, while others contributed food for the freezer. A friend occasionally left a colorful, washable nylon bag hanging on the doorknob of my back porch with helpful supplies and sometimes a welcome bottle of Chardonnay. One of these bags was always with me (without the wine) to help me stay organized. As described in the section in Chapter 2 on learning to be an advocate, the bag can contain useful items, from chargers, books, paper clips and sandwich bags to granola bars and Post-It notes.

One friend drove by as needed to let out our two dogs while I spent long hours at the hospital. Several people brought books to fill the hours of sitting around; we appreciated the choice of reading materials, including a collection of crossword puzzles and a couple of joke and riddle books that matched our corny sense of humor. A church member noticed that our gutters were full of leaves; the following week, he and a friend brought over a ladder and cleaned them out.

These were all gifts I will never forget—assurances that we were loved and that we were not facing our battles alone. They freed me to focus on my husband and his care, to be by his side without worrying about outside chores.

We can choose our own personal ways to show that we care. Even when we don't have the power to change the circumstances of others, we always have the power to be kind.

Chapter 5

Rehabilitation

All we can give back and all God wants from any of us is to humbly and proudly return the product that we have been given—which is ourselves.

Richard Rohr, *Falling Upward*

May 6, 2013
From: Kandy
Subject: It's tournament time

In a bright, clean room in a bright, clean two-story rehabilitation hospital in Charlotte, a once-busy trial lawyer, family man, and beach lover is lying in a hospital bed dreaming of going to work, cheering at a grandchild's baseball game, pulling a Spanish mackerel out of the ocean, and sharing a big slice of banana cream pie. Although the nurses and therapists are wonderful, he is tired of being helpless, tired of spending most of every day in bed, tired of being prodded and poked, tired of being hungry, and tired of boring TV that he doesn't choose to watch (very little baseball on hospital channels). He isn't *complaining much, but you know it from his eyes and his sighs. Even so, as so often happens, just when you think are getting to rock bottom, just at the right time, something good happens. Some call it luck. We call it the grace of God.*

We Cospers love sports cliches. So just when we thought he was down for the count... running out of gas on turn two... backed up at the goal line on third and fifteen... he got a pitch he could hit. He put on his game face and went out to meet the opposition. And slowly, the floppy left arm lifted to bat a balloon, and Harvey got up to walk on the parallel bars.

The hospital Care Team met today and came back to us with a projected release date of May 21 to go...home! ... with some home health care assistance. Although his recovery will take months overall, they are expecting that he will be able to use stairs by then. He will need to have his heart shocked back into rhythm and work to be able to get rid of the feeding tube. But they do feel confident he can come home successfully and safely. We have also set a goal of getting to Wilmington for a few weeks in June, where our house is more conducive to one-level living than our Charlotte home.

The sense of humor never fails. As this larger-than-life man sat at a table holding a long, thick string, struggling to use his left hand to feed the string through the holes in fat beads of red, blue, green, and yellow, "I feel like I am in preschool," he said. As he attempted to cheat by using his stronger hand, the therapist asked what he did for a living, and he said, "Lawyer." We all laughed. Then he corrected, "Professional bead-stringer."

So all the days of rain stopped this afternoon and the sun came through the windows in his room. I brought him a new cell phone and iPad so he can start feeling more connected to the outside world again. He might not be ready to throw for a touchdown or win the World Series, but he is out of pit road on the home stretch and aiming for a par on the eighteenth hole. It's a long way down the field, but we are inching toward home, a step at time. And all those cheers from all of you in the stands are giving us the support we need to get there. Go, team!

Levels of Care After the Hospital

As I emerge from the elevator and round the corner, down the long hall I can see the figure of a tall old man in a red baseball cap slumped in a wheelchair in front of the nurses' desk. The chair is too small for him; his skinny legs poke out over the footrests. He cradles his drooping head in his right hand, while his left arm dangles over the metal wheel. I draw in a quick breath as my eyes widen, then fill with tears: that figure is my husband.

This picture will remain in my memory for the rest of my life. In all the days and months to follow, I never got used to the vulnerability, the helplessness, the indignity, the falling of the mighty oak. Surely what remained of Harvey after the stroke were the truly important things: kindness, wit, intellectual curiosity, interest in other people beyond interest in himself. But for me, the specter in the red baseball cap, still the youngest and sharpest in a sea of damaged and broken bodies and minds, always took my breath away and often brought me to tears.

As I wheeled him down long tiled hallways, learned how to reposition his feet and legs in bed and readjust his pillows, heard his groans as aides struggled to transfer him from bed to chair, as I combed his hair and trimmed his mustache, as I pulled his weakened arm from the spokes of the wheelchair and fitted his bony feet into warm socks, I never got used to his dependency. It was incongruous. It didn't make sense. It made me feel sick.

An important job of hospital social workers, as part of the patient's medical team, is to help decide where patients will go next, once they are stable. The decisions are made according to the strict coverage provisions of insurance companies and Medicare, based on reports from doctors and therapists. Depending on how well they can take care of their own activities of daily living (ADL), patients can be released from the hospital to one of four types of care (these are further described in Chapter 12). Some facilities offer all or a combination of these services. Choices are as follows:

- **home,** if they are doing well enough to live there safely, with or without family companions or therapy, or if they can afford appropriate in-home care;
- **acute rehabilitation,** if they can benefit from, and physi-

cally handle, extensive rehabilitation treatment for an average of three hours per day for up to twenty-one days;
- **subacute rehabilitation,** if less aggressive therapy is warranted and they will take longer to improve, or
- **nursing home,** if they are not expected to improve.

Harvey had many problems to overcome and much work to do before he could live at home. He was exhausted, physically and emotionally. There was a lot of discussion about whether he could exert three hours a day in physical, occupational, and speech therapy. Ultimately, however, we were encouraged when he was recommended for inpatient acute rehab.

We could not have foreseen then, as he began that first stint in rehab, just how many times Harvey would need to be hospitalized and moved among all the types of available facilities. In the next two and a half years, he would go through inpatient rehabilitation six times in five different places.

Sixteen days after the stroke, though, we were still hopeful for recovery as an aide pushed his bed through a maze of hallways, elevators, and a tunnel into the rehabilitation hospital next door. The facility was clean and organized, the therapists were excellent, and the nurses were friendly. I thought, *This is going to be the place in which Harvey improves enough to go home.*

On the second morning, when I walked into the huge carpeted therapy room, I saw women and men of all ages engaged with therapists wearing scrubs. Patients were lying on wooden platforms with plastic mattresses as their arms or legs were bent and then straightened in the air. Patients slowly climbed sets of wooden steps, threw colored balls, batted balloons, balanced between parallel bars, paced on walkers and canes, pedaled stationary bikes, and strung beads. Some rested in wheelchairs while others swung in contraptions that helped them exercise.

I found Harvey seated in front of a white magnetic board. Spread on the table before him were red letters of the alphabet. The therapist was instructing him to use his good hand to line up all the letters in order. "This is a successful lawyer!" I wanted to shout. "Nineteen years of education! He was just writing briefs and interviewing witnesses. What are you people thinking?"

But I sat quietly to watch as he then crammed all the letters onto the right-hand side of the board, leaving the entire left side empty. On the table in front of him was one of the strangest clocks I had ever seen; having been asked to draw a clock face that showed the time as two o'clock, my precise husband had drawn a wobbly circle in which all of the numbers had been crowded on the right side. It was classic "left side neglect." It looked perfectly okay to him.

As the days passed, we began to see just how difficult rehabilitation would be. So many of our physical activities, so much of what our bodies can do, we take for granted when we are healthy. Yet learning to sit up, roll from side to side, balance, walk, swallow, dress, read, and write can be like marathon training for an adult with brain injury.

Beyond the physical and mental demands, the most difficult part of that first rehab—and of his many stays in medical facilities after that—was, in his words, "being tossed around like I'm in a clothes dryer." Since he could not reposition his body without help, he was uncomfortable most of the time. The yellow "FALL RISK" sign beside his door and on his hospital bracelet alerted everyone that he was not allowed out of bed unless a physical or occupational therapist was present to make sure he was moved safely—but he could not have managed to get up by himself, anyway. The therapists each came once a day, five or six days a week, for less than an hour each time; the rest of the time, he was in bed or, occasionally, propped in a recliner.

Given his height, left side weakness, lack of balance, poor physical conditioning, and tendency to faint upon standing, he needed at least two qualified people to move him. So the therapists, nurses, CNAs, and techs took care of his needs—bathing and dressing, changing sheets, administering tube feedings and medications, drawing endless vials of blood—all while he was in bed. Every time he wanted to be moved, we had to push the call button and wait our turn for the busy staff to finish helping other patients. They spent many hours trying to help him learn to use his good right hand to grab the bedrails to assist them in moving and turning him. He quickly wearied of being handled and pushed and pulled, even though there was no alternative.

All the while, everyone had to be so careful about the delicate skin on his hands and arms. It was difficult for even the gentlest of helpers to avoid tearing it. And with so many people in and out of the room, it was hard to make sure everyone knew about it. Dressings and bandages stuck to his skin. His arms and hands were always covered with purple and black splotches of various sizes and shapes.

As the rolls of white non-stick wrapping covering wounds

proliferated on his arms and legs, Harvey began to refer to himself as "the mummy." Eventually, a nurse made big pink laminated signs that read "NO TAPE ON SKIN" that I posted over his bed in every room of every hospital, rehab, and nursing home room in which he eventually stayed.

An upper arm wound from an altercation with our ficus tree back home, weeks earlier, had become infected, and it took many weeks to grow the cultures to determine what kind of germ to treat with antibiotics. As a result, we added infectious disease specialists to our long and growing list of medical friends.

Sadly, my husband became so leery of being touched that I avoided most physical contact with him except what was necessary to help. As much as I wanted us to hold each other, I settled for a quick kiss upon arriving or departing. This added to my own pain and grief.

Meanwhile, we continued to be reminded in unexpected moments that we were loved and cared for—moments of pure grace.

An Angel Visits

The days were running into one another, full of trips up and down the halls, calling for help, therapy sessions, medical procedures and tests, discussions about therapies and treatments, trying to find time to eat or get outside for a walk, responding to emails and phone calls, and, most of all, discerning Harvey's needs and how best to meet them. I was getting claustrophobic

Rehabilitation

in the elevators and the tortuous hospital parking lot.

As I walked out of the rehabilitation hospital one evening about halfway through the prescribed inpatient stay in rehab, thick clouds were blowing across the sky and thunder rumbled in the distance. Sad and frustrated, I looked up and said out loud to God, "Okay, I've had it. I need you to take it from here. I just can't do it anymore."

Looking forward to a glass of cold white wine, my lovable dogs, and my comfortable bed, I drove nearly all the way home before realizing I had left my cell phone in Harvey's room. At the last stop sign before turning onto my street, I put my head on the steering wheel and breathed a bad word. Calls and messages were coming in on that phone at all hours, including those from doctors and from our children; I had to go back. Rain spattered the windshield as I turned around and retraced my route to the parking lot, punching in the code to open the gate. I was wrapped up in my own feelings, angry with myself and with the whole situation, blind to anything but Harvey's suffering and my own exhaustion.

So when a young man called out to me as I ran through the lot in the rain, I ignored him. He caught up with me inside, at the elevator. "Mrs. Cosper. Hello. I was in school with your daughter, Ann."

I looked at the thin young man with curly hair and glasses whom I had not known well and had not seen in many years. "Oh, hi. Ann is here every weekend," I said. "Her dad is upstairs; he had a stroke. What brings you here?"

The young man hesitantly told me that he had come "to

meet with a group." Then he asked, "May I come and see Mr. Cosper?" I wasn't sure how to respond. Until that point, we had not allowed visitors. "Okay, sure," I said warily. "I'm just running back to pick up my phone."

We found Harvey lying quietly in the dark room. The young man strode forward, introduced himself, and lifted Harvey's outstretched good hand to shake it. Then he asked, "Would it be all right if I prayed for you?"

At the foot of the bed, he folded his hands, bowed his head, and stood quietly. "You can pray out loud," I said. "We are praying folks." But the young man continued to stand, still and silent, in reverent concentration. I bowed my head. Harvey closed his eyes. As minutes passed, a great tranquility spread over us. We breathed deeply. And slowly, I felt the Holy Spirit filling the room.

Finally, the young man gently reached across the bed again for Harvey's hand. "God bless you, sir," he said, and we knew that He already had.

"Young man," Harvey told him, "you can come and visit me any time."

After he left, I retrieved my phone just as it rang. It was David calling from New Zealand. Because of the time difference, he had not been able to speak with his dad very often. I laid the phone on Harvey's chest, and David said all the right things, all the meaningful things to show his understanding and love —compassionate words that I had been unable to say: "Dad, I know this is so hard for you. I know you really miss your work. You must be so frustrated. I miss you. I love you. You will get better in time."

Before they hung up, Harvey told him, "David, an angel visited me in my room tonight."

Had I not forgotten my phone, the angel would not have visited. Harvey would not have been able to talk to his son from across the globe. I later discovered that the young man had survived some tragic circumstances and struggled through a difficult recovery. God had surely appointed him an angel that night, answering our deepest prayers and bringing us a profound sense of peace.

Getting Through Long Days

For the patient, one of the most difficult parts of inpatient rehabilitation is boredom. Harvey did not feel up to entertaining many visitors; he was too uncomfortable to sleep much, and the revolving door of hospital staff performing procedures continued day and night. He did not have the interest, attention span, visual or hearing acuity for movies or television shows. The limited cable channels carried few of the sporting events that he would normally enjoy.

Graham's suggestion to **personalize the room** served not only to introduce the patient to the staff and provide conversation starters but also to provide a more pleasant and interesting environment. Even though he didn't seem to notice much about his surroundings at first, the kids and I added to the plants, flowers, and balloons from friends, decorating Harvey's room with his get-well cards, family photos, and funny posters.

The Defense Rests

We began to **listen to music** for hours. Harvey was a great lover of music, from classical to pop. He and his father had spent decades listening to Chopin, Brahms, and Beethoven, from symphonies to piano solos. He also remembered hundreds of popular songs, who wrote them and who performed them. He and David, who earned a doctorate in music and teaches university students, had spent countless happy hours in musical discussions. Harvey had cracked us up on many a long trip with his Roy Orbison imitations. To pass the long hours in bed, he lay peacefully with his eyes closed, relaxing into the sounds. Since the stroke, Harvey had difficulty with tasks such as donning headphones and managing a remote to tune into radio stations or setting his phone for playlists. David purchased some equipment to improve reception in the institutional rooms, and I always tried to leave Harvey with music playing.

Over the next two and a half years, I **read books out loud**, starting with *The Help*, moving to *The Boys in the Boat*, *Ordinary Grace*, *The Tender Bar*, *The Elephant Whisperer*, and many others. I shared my interest in novels while he shared his interest in nonfiction. To this day, a bookmark sticks up about two-thirds of the way through a biography of Charles Lindbergh that we never finished. These readings became a surprisingly fulfilling and intimate time for us.

As rehab progressed, we did begin to **accept visitors, asking them to text in advance to make sure of the timing**. Those who came at convenient times and did not stay long were most welcome distractions during the long, boring days, especially on weekends. In fact, at this point, visitors were so important in keeping Harvey's spirits up and providing mental stimulation that I began to call friends to come for visits. Most interesting during this time was seeing which people actually showed up: some with whom we had never been close became regular and most welcome visitors, while we did not see some of our closer friends. We understood that people are busy and some are uncomfortable in hospitals. We were just grateful to hear from so many folks who were cheering us on, day in and day out.

One day, during one of many hospitalizations, Harvey lay in a patterned gown on top of the sheets quietly reminiscing about his grandfather's boathouse at a lake in Georgia. For an hour or more, he described the wooden sides of the house, the boats, the rods and reels that hung on the walls. Afterwards, I encouraged him to **dictate a memoir** of his life. I regret this idea did not occur to us sooner, so that he would have time to finish it. At our request, the law firm furnished us with an app that he could use with his cell phone (with help from the speech therapist and me), sending the dictation directly for transcribing. At first he wanted to entitle it "Thirty-Eight Years at the Bar," but eventually he settled on "The Defense Rests." We ended up with fewer boyhood memories and courtroom stories than nostalgia for the cars he had driven over the years. He didn't end up with enough material for a book, but he enjoyed doing it, and our family will treasure it.

In summary, even while those long days in rehab were exhausting, boring, and scary, they were also surprisingly peaceful and intimate. As days stretched to weeks, Harvey and I continued to hope—no, expect—that eventually he would come home to a more-or-less normal, pre-stroke life. Today, reading the updates I sent to our friends at the time, I am filled with sadness and compassion for our hopeful selves.

As the prescribed three weeks of acute rehabilitation drew toward an end, even though I tried to be cheerful and positive, I knew he wasn't ready to come home. And I wasn't ready, either.

Sunday, May 19, 2013
From: Kandy
Subject: Pentecost

As I am sitting on our back porch on this Sunday morning, church bells have started to chime from somewhere in the neighborhood. "How Great Thou Art" is wafting through the damp leaves. It's Pentecost Sunday and, as churches all over the world are celebrating the arrival of the Holy Spirit in a group of grieving and unsteady believers all those centuries ago, I have to remember the promise Jesus made that he would always be with us. This happens in tiny ways in small lives every day.

If all goes well, Harvey will be home for good in two days, on Tuesday, May 21. The rehab staff tells us this is another of the miracles they often see, when someone sick and paralyzed leaves on his feet after only a few weeks. Unsurprisingly, Harvey has been very determined. He has had to learn how to sit up, walk, climb stairs one at a time, use his left leg and lift his left arm. He is still learning how to recognize things to his left, including words on a page; learning how to swallow and many other activities we all take for granted. Meanwhile,

Rehabilitation

I am learning how to coach and assist, feed him through a tube, and make a house handicap-accessible. There are some strange aluminum devices cropping up around our house and in the car. We expect the need for these to be temporary as progress continues.

We will have lots of visits from recreational, occupational, and speech therapists, nurses, and home health aides for a few weeks. We plan to be in Charlotte until mid-June, then go to our place in Wilmington (more convenient with a downstairs bedroom, and being totally up-fitted in our absence by dear friends) for a couple of weeks, while Graham and his family are in Kenya on a medical mission. We have been advised not to have visitors for the first few days at home as we get adjusted. I am sadly turning down tempting and generous offers of food for now, as Harvey is still on tube feed for another week or two. I hope not much longer - he has lost more than thirty pounds!

They say that who we really are comes out during adversity. Who Harvey really is, then, is the same as he is during good times: faithful, polite, patient, prayerful, humorous, and grateful. We thank all of you for helping him to the distinct honor of receiving the most cards of anyone our nurses have ever seen. Carolinas Rehab is a place of kind, helpful professionals who see miracles every day, and we will never forget them. Harvey calls each one by name as they come and go.

The chimes have stopped and it's time to get going for

the day. We have a long way to go and a tough road still ahead, but the worst is over. We are so excited about this homecoming and ready to get on with life, with whatever changes there will be for us. Thanks to every one of you for walking along beside us. "I shall bow in humble adoration, and there proclaim: my God, how great Thou art." Happy Pentecost!

Part 2

When Illness Becomes Disability

> *You gain strength, courage, and confidence by every experience in which you really stop to look fear in the face. You must do the things which you think you cannot do.*
> — Eleanor Roosevelt

CHAPTER 6

When Home Is Not the Same, Episode 1

Life's challenges are not supposed to paralyze you; they're supposed to help you discover who you are.

Bernice Johnson Reagon

The Wife Needs to Get a Grip

The doctor raised her voice at me in the cafeteria, but I was already crying.

Earlier that morning, she had informed us that Harvey had maximized his time in acute rehab and would be released the following week. I had three choices: take him home and care for him myself; take him home and hire some help; or, her recommendation, check him into a nursing home.

"What about more rehab?" I had pleaded. "Can't you keep him longer? Can't you refer him for more inpatient therapy so that he has more time to improve?" But she had repeated the choices; remaining at this hospital was not an option.

An hour later, she spotted me as I stood in line with my food tray, wiping tears from my face, and our eyes met. She walked over to me and said, "You need to get a grip."

"But I can't care for him at home," I said. "And I just can't put him in a nursing home!"

"Then you need to make other arrangements," she replied. We stood there for a few seconds before she turned and left.

She was a competent doctor, certainly, but she was young. She had no idea what it was like to be me: suddenly to be caring for the man you have loved and lived with and depended upon every day for more than forty years, who can no longer dress himself or walk anywhere without help. A man who needs about forty doses of medications that have to be put in meticulous order, crushed, and fed with liquid through a tube at different times each day. Who faints and falls to the floor. Who is thirteen inches taller and a hundred pounds heavier than I. Who will have to take three steps into the house and fourteen steps up to the bedroom and shower. Whose left arm dangles by his side. Who still thinks he can go to work tomorrow.

Graham told me later that he had several conversations with the doctor about his father's situation, and they knew I was resisting the obvious choice of a nursing home. In fact, I refused to consider it.

The all-business social worker had already assured me that insurance would never cover subacute rehabilitation for Harvey—more weeks in a medical institution with less intensive therapy. The patient had reached his inpatient goals, he reported, and was approved to go home. Therapists would come to the house a few times a week, he said. "Hire help if you need it." He passed along

When Home Is Not the Same, Episode 1

a list of home health agencies. Then he had handed me a list of nursing homes in the area. Not a single one had a top rating.

I had visited many times in nursing homes, or skilled nursing centers, over the years—to see relatives, friends, and church members, and to entertain the residents with singing. Both of my parents suffered extended illnesses and dementia, and both had died in a skilled nursing center—my mother at the age of seventy-seven, ten years prior to Harvey's illness, and my father at the age of eighty-seven, just two years before Harvey's stroke. A nursing home did not seem the right place for a competent sixty-four-year-old professional who was going to get well and return to work. Reluctantly, though, I had taken the list and inspected the highest-rated facility in our area of town. It was old and dated, with stained linoleum floors and battered walls. Wheelchairs littered the long hallways. Women and men with wispy gray hair leaned on bony arms, their shriveled legs dangling over the footrests. Bathroom and disinfectant smells filled the air. Televisions blared. Each small green-painted room held two hospital beds a few feet apart, a straight wooden chair, and a metal table. Harvey would be twenty-five years younger than most of the residents. He would have no privacy and little quiet. He would lie in bed most of the time.

As my heart filled with compassion for the people living there and for their families, I felt nauseated. Trying to picture Harvey there was like trying to fit a piece into the wrong puzzle. I could only imagine the emotional damage that would cause while he worked toward—and hoped for—recovery.

He will be miserable, I thought; *he will give up, and he will die in here.* I got back into my car and cried all the way back to the hospital.

I was surprised that Harvey, even with the flat emotional affect the stroke had caused, had not been begging to go home. I think he knew how difficult it would be, and how much assistance he still needed. He also seemed more depressed and less willing to fight for himself. Meanwhile, I felt sick at the thought of trying to care for him by myself. Around-the-clock care would cost at least twenty dollars an hour, seven days a week: nearly fourteen thousand dollars a month! *Who could afford that?* Disability payments would eventually run out. And even if we could afford some help for a while, who would we hire? How much time would they spend sitting around the house when we didn't need them? Where would they sleep? Wouldn't they still need a second person—me—to help him move around, to get him off the floor when he fell?

This happens to families every day: disabled loved ones leaving the hospital are given lists of residential care facilities and home health agencies, and they have no idea what to do. They are making painfully life-altering decisions, trying to balance the financial implications with what is best for the patient and everyone else involved. Sometimes there seem to be no good choices.

The loss of income because of illness and disability can be catastrophic, forcing families to make impossible choices. What about those for whom disability insurance is not an option? When a young breadwinner suddenly loses the ability to live an independent life? When the family will lose its ability to pay the bills if a parent quits a job to become a full-time caregiver for a sick spouse or child? When the sick person has been living from paycheck to paycheck? When frail elderly people deplete their savings and have to sell everything of value they own? In trying to decide what to do at this point, I was fully aware that, even though our situation was tough, we were not yet struggling with financial imperatives that many others must face right away. And it has certainly influenced my views in the ongoing national debate about the government's role in health care, including Medicaid and Medicare.

Thanks to a decision Harvey was fortunate to be able to make years earlier, we had more choices than many people have. For years, while supporting our family and trying to save for retirement, he had elected to pay high premiums for disability insurance. With the exception of some freelance projects, I had been a stay-at-home mom, and the five of us had depended on his ability to work. The policy would provide short-term and, if needed, long-term disability income for several years before we would have to begin depleting our retirement savings and investments, which included our home and the house at the coast. As it turned out, paying those disability premiums over the years was a fortuitous decision, and we were glad Harvey had been able to afford them through the law firm.

Dependent upon the periodic doctors' reports, Harvey's policy provided us with a monthly disability check that we were able to spend in the ways we needed it most for a period of several years. In the end, he would not need the insurance for as long as it would have paid out.

After the doctor chastised me in the cafeteria, I decided

to call a home health agency on the social worker's list. I contracted out-of-pocket for three eight-hour shifts of help for the first few days at home, at twenty dollars per hour. The aide on the first shift would ride with me to the hospital to help bring Harvey home. I feared it would not go well.

May 23, 2013
Ann's Facebook Post

    Ready or not, Dad comes home today, after forty days in the hospital. We are nervous but excited to have him back in the beautiful home he and my mom have worked to create over many years, which will be full of contractors and therapists coming in and out to make sure the house is safe for Dad. Please pray that their home is a safe place that will be an impetus for Dad's continued recovery. Please pray for strength, grace, and the ability to know God's love and see God's work for my incredible mom, who is at once a sacrificial and loving wife, general contractor, physical therapist, nursemaid, housekeeper, bookkeeper, cheerleader, dog owner, errand boy, caregiver, companion, and, still, a concerned mother and friend. As you can imagine, this is uncharted territory for us, so it is hard to anticipate what we will need when. Simply being available when we need you is the best thing you can do for our family right now, keeping in mind that this may mean dropping what you're doing to help out. Mom is overrun with calls scheduling appointments, directing people, etc., but if you want to help and really mean it, I am sure we could use it. I will be home in Charlotte this weekend, so instead of contacting her, please contact me. Message me for my phone number if you need it. We appreciate so much your continued prayers and support. Today brings new challenges, so keep sending 'em up for the big guy, his saint of a wife, and everyone who is assisting in up-fitting Mom and Dad's houses and helping Dad regain strength and function.

- On his post-fall appearance: "I look like I've been through a meat grinder."

- On his compression socks: "All I'm missing is a garter belt."

Thanks for your continued support and prayers for him and my incredible, resilient, tireless, devoted mom.

The Deepest Part of the Ocean

On Thursday, May 23, after forty days in various parts of the hospital, Harvey was released to go home. On rolling carts, we arranged the flowers, plants, cards, posters, reading glasses, hearing aids, baseball caps, instructions, prescriptions, unworn clothes, and leftover supplies. The aide from the home health agency and several nurses helped us load everything into my old black SUV. From our church lending closet, I had gratefully borrowed a used portable wheelchair.

A few minutes into the twelve-minute ride home, Harvey announced that he had to go to the bathroom. I told him he had to wait. He said it again. I told him he had to wait. When we drove up the driveway, the aide and I threw open the car doors. We grabbed the walker and tried to help Harvey out of the car without bumping his head or falling, sliding his heavy left leg and arm as we went. You can't rush a person who is recovering from a stroke. The dogs ran outside and waggled underfoot as we helped him up the three steps.

As soon as the aide maneuvered Harvey through the kitchen and into the bathroom, I heard a loud crash, then a sickening thud. Bleeding from several places on his arms and legs, Harvey lay scrunched on the floor between a crushed wicker basket and the toilet. We could not figure out how to get him up. He had been home for less than five minutes.

Fortunately, the preceding day, some friends had helped me round up bedding parts to set up a small cot in our den. It was intended to be a temporary resting place during the day before he went upstairs to sleep at night in our room. The aide and I managed, after about twenty minutes, to help maneuver his lanky body from the bathroom floor and into that little bed. As his legs protruded from above the ankle on the short mattress, and his elbows poked out the sides, we would ordinarily have found the picture comical—only this time, we didn't laugh.

The garage renovation was still in the planning stages, and it was obvious that Harvey was not going to make the trip upstairs to our bedroom, not any time soon. We were going to need a hospital bed. As the clock neared 5:00 p.m. on his first day home, I called home health suppliers until I found one that could deliver a bed the next day. When the medical equipment

When Home Is Not the Same, Episode 1

company phoned on Saturday morning at 7:00 to say they were on the way, I had to awaken neighbors to come over and help me dismantle the cot to make room.

Harvey tried. We all tried. But, over the next three days, he toppled over with every caregiver who came, at every shift, whenever he tried to get out of bed. There was blood on sheets, carpets, and clothing. We called 911 more than once for medics to help us get him up. I borrowed a bedside commode from the church closet. I was the only person allowed to administer his tube feeds and meds, for which the scheduling was as complicated to me as computer programming. Thankfully, Lisa had sorted the first rounds of pills into an organizer for me. As I crushed and funneled them into his belly every four hours, the fortified solution caused severe diarrhea. The caregivers called up the stairs or rang the cell phone beside my pillow at all hours of the night to help get Harvey off the floor. Since our downstairs rooms all open onto each other, I hesitated to prepare food in the kitchen so that Harvey wouldn't be sad at smelling or seeing real food, which he had been denied for many weeks. We ate surreptitiously, putting together sandwiches or salads while he was napping.

Thank goodness Ann had made yet another trip home from Raleigh. She was the one bright spot of that horrible weekend. She knew that her visits brought joy and hope to both her father and me. She engaged her dad in games to stretch his mind and exercise his weak left hand. She kept his mind active with legal questions from her own work, as well as from the cases he had managed. But Ann was living and working in a city three hours away and, behind her cheerful smile and ever-present humor, we knew, she was hurting and exhausted and under pressure to attend to her job, as were her brothers. Graham was on call at the hospital, operating on children day and night, while trying to spend time with his wife and children. David was teaching hundreds of students at a university across the globe.

We were concerned for all three children, as they were concerned for their dad and me. They loved and supported us in their own precious ways, but they couldn't be present every day to help out at home. We would never have wanted them to. They had their own busy lives to live. Somehow we had to figure out a different plan. Harvey didn't seem interested in making decisions, and he acquiesced to my judgment. As his illness morphed into disability, I felt the weight of so many responsibilities and wondered constantly whether I was doing the right thing—if there was a "right" thing.

Although he was unable to do anything but lie on the cot, I don't remember that Harvey complained that weekend, not once. But I knew that being home was not what he had expected; we both knew that he was not safe.

Two disastrous days after the start of that first stint at home, I tried to control my panic as I contacted the social worker from rehab—the one who had assured me Harvey would neither need nor qualify for more inpatient rehab. I asked the man for a list of all the subacute rehabs in our area. Then I researched them online. A friend who was an experienced parish nurse put me in touch with a social worker at what she judged to be one of the best facilities in town, and I called to make an impassioned plea to have Harvey admitted there as soon as possible. It was Memorial Day weekend, which complicated the planning.

Finally, we received the news that Asbury, the rehabilitation section of the Aldersgate Methodist retirement complex, had a room available. I made the decision to move him, despite not having visited the place and not knowing whether our health insurance would cover it.

The next day, I was thankful to learn that, in spite of what I had been told, the stay would indeed be covered by insurance for up to twenty-one days, as long as therapists confirmed that the patient was making progress. Harvey would participate in physical, occupational, and speech (swallowing) therapy while living in a large private room with twenty-four-hour nursing care. Such a relief. Those four days at home will always be among the worst memories of my life.

May 25, 2013
From: Kandy
Subject: The Deepest Part of the Ocean

Ann is standing beside Harvey's hospital bed in our den as they are lifting weights with their left hands - his weight is one pound and hers is five pounds. They are up to thirty reps already. Our caregiver this shift - an Army sergeant who is kind, professional, and just what the "old man" needs - is patiently waiting for the next load of laundry to be done, the next small need of her tall, now-skinny patient to be expressed. I am preparing to give him another of his every-four-hours tube feedings.

The trip home on Thursday was overly eventful, ending with a fall on weakened knees in the bathroom with a well-intended male caregiver. This has been followed by several more falls, including an eventful landing that required EMT trucks screaming to the house. As they were putting Harvey back in bed, one of the medics asked him the oft-repeated questions of what is your name, birthday, who is the president, and so on. Then the medic asked, "What is the deepest place in the ocean?" Harvey immediately responded, to which the man threw up his hands and exclaimed, "You are only the second person who has ever gotten that right in all the years I have been a medic!" Harvey hasn't lost any of his wits. Every time I pour in his latest tube feed, he says, "Sorry to be eating in front of you all."

After several days at home, it is obvious that Harvey will be safer and improve faster in another rehab facility, a highly rated part of the Methodist group. They are going to pick him up on Monday afternoon and focus on getting him stronger, especially in walking, managing stairs, and swallowing. We are all happy with this decision. It's not easy being at home when home is the same but you are different. He wants to come home when he is able to eat, navigate stairs, and participate in other normal activities.

The night before Harvey left the hospital this week, I returned to his room from our seven-year-old grandson's last baseball game of the season—just one more thing his Grin-daddy had to miss. As I sat down to boast about the big home run, Harvey said quietly, "I was just lying here thinking about how lucky we are." Then we talked about all the blessings we have. And that includes all of you and the love you have shown us. That's just who he is.

Harvey is lying here now talking about all the fish he has yet to catch in Masonboro Sound, and we hold out that hope and expectation. Thank you for your continued prayers during our journey.

P.S. The deepest place in the ocean is the bottom. Although Harvey also knew where the deepest bottom was, and how deep.

Chapter 7

Another Chance to Prepare for Home

It's okay to feel Not Very Okay At All. It can be quite normal, in fact. And all you need to do, on those days when you feel Not Very Okay At All, is come and find me, and tell me. Don't ever feel like you have to hide the fact you're feeling Not Very Okay At All. Always come and tell me. Because I will always be there.

       A. A. Milne, *Winnie-the-Pooh* (Piglet to Pooh)

May 29, 2013
From: Kandy
Subject: Moving again, taking one day at a time
  As we neared Asbury yesterday afternoon, we passed a little church with a sign out front: "One day at a time." It reminded us of a funny banner that Ann made to go on Harvey's wall. In the "Pink Panther" movie series, after the bumbling detective Clouseau has driven him crazy, former Chief Inspector Dreyfus tells his psychiatrist that he is getting "better and better—every day and in every way."

Our medical staff all recognized the allusion and laughed with us. Because, of course, as soon as Dreyfus walks out onto the grounds of the "lunatic asylum," Clouseau drives him crazy again; Dreyfus steps on a rake and knocks himself into a pond. As we drove farther on, past the guard gate, and wound our way through lovely woods to Asbury Care Center, Harvey said, "I feel like I need a rake."

Our three-car caravan (Graham, Ann with her dog, and the two of us) arrived and settled Harvey into a large, private, Carolina blue room ("although my nurses are Duke fans") with large windows. He received a warm welcome and feels quite at home now, especially since he can get more sports programs on cable TV.

After several days at home that we never want to repeat, today has been the best since the stroke. I pushed him in the wheelchair around the gardens and grounds; then we played ball, read the newspaper out loud, and Harvey successfully stacked colored cones in the therapy room using BOTH hands. ("It's sad. I am back in preschool and I feel like a mullet.") Under the watchful eye of the speech therapist, he tasted lemon pudding and some thickened iced tea, all the while wondering if steak and pot roast could be served pudding-style, and if the thickener would work on scotch or beer. Except for the times that medicines make him feel sick, and soreness from his falls interferes with his movement, Harvey is working hard and improving. We know that he is in the right place. It actually takes me less time to get there. He

Another Chance to Prepare for Home

can have visitors, especially on the slow weekends.

We never really understood just how devastating a stroke can be—what it can take away from you and how hard it is to get those things back. But they ARE coming back. Progress doesn't come fast or easily. However, there are good things, too. For instance, there has not been one mail delivery since the Monday after the stroke, six weeks ago, without at least one card, and for these expressions of caring we are so grateful. THANK YOU especially for your prayers. As we were watching the Covenant church service by computer at home on Sunday morning, we heard Harvey's name lifted in prayer, along with thanks for caregivers. In her chair there in our den, our caregiver at the time teared up along with the rest of us.

He might not be home in time for his sixty-fifth birthday on June 13, but we will have a lot to celebrate, anyway. Every day and in every way. One day at a time.

Flagging in our Zeal

"Subacute rehab" turned out to be "nursing home with some therapy, with the chance of going home eventually." In many of these facilities, patients working to regain the ability to live at home share the same floors, exercise rooms, dining facilities, and gathering spaces as those who live there permanently. Once again, Harvey was younger and more alert than most of the other patients around him, and it was less depressing for him to stay in his room than to sit among ninety-year-old dementia patients. He still wasn't eating and he was still difficult to move, although the standing and walking were indeed getting better. I took videos of his progress in the hallways and the sunny therapy room with its wall of windows. I felt renewed hope that we might have a good life ahead of us at home after all.

As we learned the first time he had tried to come home, however, we would need to make the house handicap-accessible. Even though Harvey was making progress with sets of low practice stairs, for instance, we couldn't be sure when, if, or for how long he would be able to manage our stairs at home. Our bathroom fixtures were the wrong height for a disabled person and the shower had no railings. The doorways were too narrow for a wheelchair. The edges of rugs could cause falls.

I hired the contractor who had, just a year earlier, opened up the back of our thirty-year-old house with a new kitchen and covered porch. We had decided then that there was no feasible place to add a downstairs bedroom "in case we happened to need it later, in our old age," so we opted for a modernized living space. Now the need for downstairs accommodations was real. We had to rule out the idea of a stair lift or elevator for architectural reasons. So, in between the six or seven hours a day that I spent with Harvey at rehab, I began working on plans to use the payments from his disability policy to convert the only logical remaining space—our garage—into a handicap-accessible bedroom and bathroom. A designer friend assisted with planning the space and selecting furniture, carpet, tile, and fixtures. The space would not be adequate as a master bedroom, but we would find a way to make the situation work for us.

This meant cleaning out a garage that had collected the junk of a family of five for nearly thirty years, and it meant having a storage shed built in the back yard to hold that junk. On a sweltering hundred-degree day, three dear friends showed up at the house and sent me on to Harvey's bedside at the hospital. Then they cleaned out the entire garage and storage room, organizing the new shed with all the rakes, coolers, folding chairs, tools, basketballs, hoses, sleds, planters, and paint cans. And I hadn't even asked them to come: when they heard about the plans, they just called to say they'd be there.

The new room would not be completed before Harvey was scheduled to come home, but I could drive him four hours to our Wilmington house where, with a few minor changes for accessibility, we could live on one floor. The coast would be just the place, I thought, for peaceful healing.

Once again, I was being optimistic to a fault. There would be more emergencies before we could get there, and even more after we arrived. The worst was yet to come.

June 5, 2013
Ann's Facebook Post
#dadquotes

   My dad's sixty-fifth birthday is June 13. I have decided that for the month of June I will post at least one quote from him every day. So, for June 1-5:

    - Re: being in a room full of opposing counsel: "I felt about as welcome as a turd in a punchbowl."

- On the annoyances of life: "I feel like I'm being nibbled to death by ducks."
- On having a lot to do at work: "I'm just trying to keep the snakes in their baskets."
- Me, while watching football: "Dad! We scored!" Dad: "The other team must've pulled all their players off the field." #dadquote #unclife
- On a certain college football team: "They're good. You wouldn't think so. Someone called in a bomb scare to the library and the first twenty guys out made the team."
- To a family friend pregnant with twin girls: "You should name them 'Cash' and 'Credit'."

June 8, 2013
From: Kandy
Subject: The last miles are the hardest

    Eight weeks ago tonight, life in the Cosper household took a dramatic turn when a blood clot the size of a BB shot up from Harvey's heart to his brain. Since then, he has spent fifty-four days and nights in five different rooms in three medical institutions with more than a hundred different caregivers. He has had scores of tests, procedures, examinations, and therapy sessions. He has had to relearn how to sit up, walk, use his left leg and arm, recognize things on his left side, and read. So it's understandable that, today, he is so very tired. And, having spent the greatest percentage of each day with him, with so much to

Another Chance to Prepare for Home

handle there and at home, so am I.

The good news is that there has been a lot of progress this week in all of those skills. Harvey is walking a very long way on the walker and riding an exercise bike. He is using his left arm more and more. His heart rhythm is stable. The bad news is that he had some residual infections and he still is not allowed to eat or drink independently. The bolus feedings are not satisfying to someone who dreams about fresh vegetables and barbecue, sweet tea, and cold beer. He has lost exactly forty pounds as of today.

Weekends are slow and tough, and we have needed extra strength to get through this one. Next week is full of more therapy sessions and doctor appointments. And on Thursday, there won't be any birthday cake to celebrate his sixty-fifth.

But all in all, he is progressing so well that we hope he will be home in a couple of weeks. We are converting our garage into a downstairs bedroom in case it's needed (which means building a storage building in the back yard, which means having some trees cut down, and that's the way it goes! Much to do, as always). Thanks to all of you for your continued love shown to us in so many different, helpful, and creative ways. You will never know how much it means to us.

Graham's family came yesterday with gifts, cards—the homemade ones from the grandchildren are the best!—balloons and farewells, because, as I write this, they are crossing the ocean on a long flight to Africa. We *ask for your prayers for them as Graham will be operating on children and training surgeons in Kijabe, Kenya for the next three weeks as part of a Christian doctors' initiative, while the rest of the family volunteers in an orphanage. Please pray for the patients, for their safety, and for their witness to the love of God in that part of the world.*

And pray for us, as we make the last long, difficult strides toward getting back to our own home and to a new normal, whatever that may be for us. On Sunday, elders from Covenant came out to serve us communion, but Harvey couldn't take anything by mouth, of course. So they gently held the bread and juice to his lips. We were amazed at the strength in his voice when he said the Lord's Prayer with us afterward. We were reminded, as always, how truly blessed we are, and how deeply loved.

June 12, 2013
Ann's Facebook Post
#dadquote

- Before I started law school: "Don't go to law school to do justice. Law and justice are not the same thing."
- On being useful around the house: "I can fix everything but a broken heart."
- On taking disco lessons with Mom in the seventies: "I resembled something out of a Maytag box. The instructor told me I looked like a dancing refrigerator."
- (okay, more like a scenario, from a year before the

stroke): Cosper siblings and Dad are sitting on the patio smoking cigars (nobody ever inhaled) and enjoying adult beverages. Kandy Cosper is in the house cooking dinner when she suddenly runs out waving a dish towel and screaming, "The casserole caught fire!! The house is on fire!!" and then runs back inside. Dad takes a long pull on his cigar, taps the ashes into the ashtray, and lays the cigar down. As he gets up, he says, "Excuse me. The house is on fire." And then he calmly goes inside.
- Me: "Dad, you've lost weight!" Dad: "Yeah, it's like throwing a deck chair off the Titanic."

June 13, 2013
Ann's Facebook Post

Today is my dad's sixty-fifth birthday. At 12:30 a.m., I texted him the following: "Allow me to be the first to wish you happy birthday! Sixty-five years ago, the best man in the world was born, who would love and inspire everyone he met. You are the world's best man, father, lawyer, and friend. I am so proud and so grateful for being able to call you my father. You are an inspiration. I love you!!"

I asked my mom today whether Dad got my text. Mom: "Yes. Dad said you must have been drinking."

Happy birthday to the one and only Harvey Lindenthal Cosper, Jr.!

The Defense Rests

Birthday meltdown

June 13, 2013
From: Kandy
Subject: Sick birthday

This is to let you know that Harvey is back in the hospital in Progressive Care with atrial fibrillation and a spreading infection. He is under quarantine. He will want to have visitors again once he gets back to rehab, and we will keep you posted. Harvey says this has certainly been a birthday to remember. Thanks for the cards—they are the highlight of each day, along with our daily calls from each of the kids. The Kenyan contingent reports monkeys on the roof.

Harvey's sixty-fifth birthday was another day that I will never forget. Because his heart had lapsed back into a-fib despite medication, he was scheduled to be transported to a suburban hospital for the day so that his cardiologist could shock it back into rhythm. Early that morning, when I parked at Asbury to board the wheelchair transportation van with him, I could tell he was quite ill. After he was strapped and locked into the back of the brown van, I climbed up front with the driver.

When we arrived, aides helped Harvey into a patterned gown and, painfully, onto a hospital bed. The cardiologist, who had been his friend and doctor for many years, stepped past the curtain in the waiting area. My husband felt clammy and was burning with fever. Apparently, the festering wound on his arm was spreading infection into his body. "Harvey is sick," I told him. "Is it still safe to do the procedure?"

The doctor checked the chart, examined Harvey, then shook his head: there would be no jump-starting of his heart that day. The staff called for an ambulance to transfer him to the main hospital uptown.

From inside a tiny curtained cubicle, we heard carts rattling, machines beeping, stretchers rolling, patients moaning, family members complaining, medical staff giving orders. There, on his birthday, bored, exhausted, depressed, sick and in pain, unable to eat or drink, Harvey lay quietly as five more hours ticked by. We didn't talk much—what was there to say? He couldn't concentrate on listening to a book. Finally, by mid-afternoon, an ambulance became available, and aides came to roll him away. I had to call the transportation service to take me back to Asbury for my car before heading to the hospital downtown. The brown van arrived for me after the ambulance left with Harvey on a stretcher. I was unable to muster much conversation with the driver during the ride back.

That was just one of many trips to the Emergency Department. Just one of many ambulance rides and scores of days in the hospital that were adding up over several years. Most of the others blur in my memory. But the images from that day are strong and stark. It was a day of realizing we were in it for the long haul. The road would be hard, full of detours and accidents. Somehow, we would need to find the strength to make it through.

As I drove back to the downtown hospital that summer afternoon, dark clouds hovered and rain began to pour. Once again, I rolled down my window to inform the attendant in the Emergency parking lot that my husband was being delivered by ambulance. Once again, I circled the crowded lot to find a parking spot. But this time, I didn't jump from the car and sprint toward the entrance. In fact, I couldn't get out of the car at all; I couldn't go into the hospital. I was surprised to realize that the tears on my face were not so much from sadness as from anger. Lightning and thunder shot through the air as rain and then large hail pelted my windshield. I slammed the steering wheel with my fists, shouting, "I can't do it! I can't go back into that place. I can't do this again!"

We extroverts cannot stay alone with our thoughts for long, and it often takes talking to another person to help us figure out what we're feeling. Within minutes, I had collected myself enough to press the speed dial icon on my cell phone for my closest friend since Miss Showalter's second grade at Irving Park School in Greensboro. I remembered the pink quilted bedspreads in my friend's childhood bedroom, her mother's green ceramic plates piled with fried chicken and mashed potatoes and gravy, my ukulele tuned with her piano for "Michael, Row the Boat Ashore." We knew almost everything about each other. Now a hospice supervisor with a Master of Social Work degree, also a caregiver for a sick husband, also a Christian, she always knew just how to listen, what to say, what not to say, what to ask, and what not to ask. I always feel safe with her. She answered the call.

After a few minutes of her calm, reflective listening, and our talking about how hard life can be—I think she cried, too, on her end of the call—we started laughing at the ridiculously melodramatic coincidence of a violent storm as backdrop to my personal storm. We realized that it sounded like one of those maudlin stories we so seriously wrote for Mrs. Crisp's seventh grade English class. I had famously written about Laura, a homeless, lame, orphaned little girl who wandered through foggy cobblestone streets seeking the grave of her brother, who had been trampled by horses while leaning over to pick up one of her fallen crutches. As Laura gave up trying to find the graveyard, slumped against a fence, and died alone in the darkness, a three-legged dog licked her face as, "just around the corner, the cemetery keeper clanged shut the iron gates and went home to supper."

Suddenly I was Laura, and we howled with laughter at our teenaged selves and our grown-up situations. No, I decided: I refuse to expire against the fence. After we finally hung up, I stuffed my old striped handkerchief into my bag, groped for my spiny purple umbrella, and power-walked through the rain to the ED to find my husband, who needed me.

June 14-16, 2013
Ann's Facebook Posts
#dadquote
   -Upon seeing Dad in his hospital room:
    Me: "Hey, Dad! You look great!"
    Dad: "I look like a beached whale."
   -"You get your wide hips from me. Everything else you get from your mother."
   -Me: "Sorry I'm late, but I had to get a new cover for my duvet."

> *Dad: "I don't know what a duvet is, but, as your father, I am glad to hear you're keeping it covered."*

Playing Keep-Away

The following day, when I drove out to Asbury to pick up a few things from Harvey's room, I found balloons and flowers left by friends who had visited on his birthday without knowing that he was hospitalized again. I also discovered an unwelcome present on his bed: a notice that, as of that day, he was no longer covered by insurance for subacute rehab. Based on therapists' notes, the insurance provider had determined that he had reached a plateau in his progress and would not benefit from more time in the facility. When I sought out the social worker, she explained that we could stay longer at our own expense—about $250 a day. Perhaps the few hours of daily therapy would be covered by insurance, but the room and nursing services definitely would not.

Once again, I thought, how could this man come home? Were we really that much more able to handle his living at home than we had been that disastrous Memorial Day weekend several weeks earlier? As yet, construction had barely started on our "handicap suite." He still could not eat or drink. He was walking gingerly with a cane, yes, but often fainting and falling. He could never be left alone; even when tucked safely in bed, he might not recognize the danger of trying to get up by himself, especially if he needed to get to the bathroom. How many hours of help per day could we afford to hire after paying the cost of the new room? Wouldn't we still need two people just to transfer him? I filled out the paperwork to appeal the insurance ruling. I began lining up doctors and nursing home staff to speak on his behalf when the telephone hearing would take place.

Harvey was in the hospital for five more days, during which time I paid out-of-pocket the daily rate to hold his room at Asbury. Once he was transported back there, I continued to pay for four weeks more, until he was finally released to come home—because our appeal was denied. In a cheery group email during that time, I reported that things seemed to be going better, at last.

June 23, 2013
From: Kandy
Subject: Words of the week (weak)
Pancakes!

That was the first thing Harvey asked for in the ICU after his stroke. Coincidentally (or not), it was the first thing served to him last Wednesday when, after five tries, he finally did well enough on the swallowing test to qualify for small bites of real food once a day, under supervision. The picture of his syrupy smile is going to be an all-time favorite in the family album.

Improvements

With IV medications, Harvey's heart finally converted to sinus rhythm, and his arms and throat began to heal. I was able to drive him by our house so that he could see the construction in progress: the garage that is turning into a bedroom. Now he is back at Asbury Care Center and much improved. He is benefitting from therapy to increase his strength. He looks and seems more and more like his old self.

Paperwork

The insurance company is telling us we have to go home, but we can't manage by ourselves at home yet. Harvey had another fall two nights ago, thankfully without injury. We know that he needs more practice with everyday activities. We will see what the coming week brings. Today I was sitting in his room filling out disability forms when I came across a page—one inadequate single page—for listing his doctors and medications. He suggested that I just paste in the pages of the local medical society roster, or attach the county medical directory.

Angels

My busy sister, Jan, a lawyer for the N.C. legislature, took two days off from work this week to come down and keep an eye on Harvey so that I could get some time away after months of full-time caregiving. I was able to attend the N.C. Bar Association annual meeting in Asheville as a guest of daughter Ann, who was honored as a graduate of the bar's Leadership Academy. Thank you for your prayers for Graham's family as they finish their last week as missionaries in Kenya; they call almost every day. We speak with David in New Zealand at least twice a week as he grades exams, reorganizes the music theory curriculum, and prepares to teach a new course on the Blues.

"My illness has been a good thing for the greeting card companies," Harvey says. *Every time we reach a low point and need encouragement, or help with something, God sends us angels: to clean out the garage, slip food into the refrigerator, call with a friendly message, send a kind or funny card, pop in at Asbury, email a word of cheer, leave a bag on the porch, or say a prayer for us during these hard days. We feel your prayers and thank you so much. We are the beneficiaries of so much that is good, and we are very grateful.*

June 15-26, 2013
Ann Facebook Posts
#dadquotes

- On his pale legs: "I look like I've been living under a Band-Aid."
- "The law is all about sense and touch."
- Me: "Dad, did you get a haircut?"
  Dad: "Yep, I got all of 'em cut."
- Re: getting on the scale: "It said, 'one at a time, please.'"
- On falling on Saturday morning (he's fine, fortunately): "The bigger they are, the harder they fall."
- On hoping for my future husband: "You wait for the man who puts you first, before anything else."
- Nursing home staff member: "Is this your daughter?"
  Dad: "Yep, the only one anybody talks about anyway."
- On lying diagonally in bed: "I'm a crooked lawyer."
- Several years ago, hanging up the phone after learning

that my seventy-seven-year-old grandfather (Dad's father, a retired lawyer, who is now deceased) had been apprehended for parking his giant lavender Cadillac in a fire lane in front of a department store around noon while my grandmother was shopping inside. He decided to crack open a cold case of Coors Light he just had purchased. Granddaddy offered the cop a beer. After asking how old he was, the cop said, "...I can't arrest you. Please just move your vehicle out of the fire lane." Then he went into the mall to have my grandmother paged. My dad's response: "Well, your grandfather's been on a one-man crime spree."

- Another law firm's HR director: "We're calling you to see if you know (name given)." Dad: "No, I don't know him."

HR director: "Really? He says you two were in the same fraternity in college."

Dad: "Oh, you're talking about Toad? TOAD! Yeah, Toad's great."

June 30, 2013
Ann's Facebook Post

Well, folks, last day of Dad Quote Month. There are SO many others, and bear in mind that there are others that are probably offensive to most people and therefore could not be put on here. Anyway, I leave you with the following from today:

- "Look at my skinny legs. Yours are better. Yours have

more meat on them. Mine look like something a bird should be on top of."
- Me: "Dad, I've seen the pictures of you and mom in college in your little tennis hotpants."
Dad: "Yes. That was when men were men and shorts were shorts."
- Me: "Dad, don't you miss Hank (dachshund nemesis at home)?"
Dad: "Yeah, like a toothache."

Finally we were able to make a plan for Harvey to graduate from rehab for what we believed would be the final time. But once again, you can see from my emails that our plans were optimistic, at best. It turned out that we were just playing keep-away, after all.

July 2, 2013
From: Kandy
Subject: Playing keep-away
    Remember that game in which someone reaches out to give you something and, just when you stretch out your hand for it, they snatch it away? It makes babies laugh. But it can make adults cry.
    This week, knowing that we were fighting the puzzling coverage denials of insurance for rehab, along with our deep weariness of institutional living, we planned a clean getaway to Wilmington for this coming Friday. We sent down food and supplies with loyal friends. We arranged

to have family waiting for us. But then...the good staff here paid us a visit. They said that their policy was to discharge rehab patients when they reach a plateau; that Harvey was still making a good recovery, and that he was working hard enough to merit more time with their therapists. So he is being rewarded for his progress by the opportunity to stay longer and do even better. (Now we just need to convince the insurance company of this.) It was one of those sad, happy moments that seem to come almost every day now.

So we're still here in rehab. The work continues, with renewed hope, a vow to fight exhaustion, and a smattering of real joy. Today Harvey practiced walking up flights of stairs. Today we took ourselves to the barber shop. He told the barber, "When your hair stops growing on your head, it starts coming out of your ears and nose." Today the eye doctor prescribed glasses that will help with the deficit in peripheral vision. Graham and the children, safely back from Kenya, came to visit, bubbling with stories of baboons, zebras, friendly African children, long plane rides, successful surgeries and training of Kenyan surgeons, and a cat that ate the mice in their house there. Today Harvey ate three full meals: scrambled eggs and sausage, turkey and rice, stuffed pepper and vanilla pudding. (Still no thin liquids, so still the tube for water and medications.) Today we read out loud to each other and prayed over supper together in his room. There was so much to be thankful for.

Another Chance to Prepare for Home

Tonight, on the eighty-first evening since the stroke, he is watching the Braves from his bed at Asbury while I watch with my bowl of popcorn at home. I try not to be sad that his favorite chair here is still empty, because I know he is getting better, "every day and in every way." The neurologist who examined him recently could tell that Harvey was okay when they were talking about what Harvey did for a living (doctors really like hearing this, though most of them have already heard of him, if not been defended by him) and what kind of challenge to his brain that kind of work is. The doctor mentioned politicians and Harvey said, "I wouldn't need a brain for that."

If I haven't responded to your call, email, note, or kind gesture, please forgive me. With our house under construction, I am overwhelmed with decisions: what kind of toilet do you want? Tile, carpet, and where do you want outlets, and what size should we make the closet? Our builder is making it easier than it could be. Meanwhile, I am dealing with applications for disability and COBRA; sending endless faxes and phone messages; trying to "exercise and eat right and get plenty of sleep," while spending six to eight hours per day at Aldersgate; checking on Harvey's medications and progress; and keeping up with so many wonderful, loyal friends who, like God, "will never leave you alone."

I could write a book about all the ways God has loved us through this, through our incredible friends. And last weekend, Ann actually counted Harvey's basket of cards, topping 400! (Yes, it can get boring in rehab, and we look for diversions.) We enjoy reading cards every night. Thank you so much for your love, visits, constancy, encouragement, prayers, and faith. One day, we will be back out in the world with you, with the great privilege of doing for others what has been done for us. Of being there for you when something you reached for is taken away. Because there is always going to be something else to reach for—something good.

July 5, 2013
From: Kandy
Subject: Lucky 13

Exactly 13 weeks after his stroke on April 13, Harvey Cosper is making his escape from living in medical institutions. He is coming on home on Saturday, July 13. Harvey was born on June 13.

All you triskaidekaphobians can make of that what you will. We believe in luck, both good and bad. But mostly we believe in blessings. We believe in the love of God, directly and through others, to carry us through all the good and bad luck in life. What we see now is simply a determined man who hit a bad spot in the road and, aided by the medical community and countless acts of love and kindness, began to overcome the tremendous challenges he has faced.

Early in his career, when he became exposed to so much that is disappointing and negative and mean in the world, Harvey had an older lawyer/mentor say to him: "Cosper, people are just no damn good." But yesterday, acknowledging the smiles and congratulations of the staff as he trekked for the hundredth time down the Aldersgate halls on his well-worn walker, Harvey said, "I am going to have to recant all those times that I repeated that quote."

During the extra week in rehab, Harvey has made excellent progress. My crazy sister and her husband came for a welcomed visit and we actually took him out to lunch twice. It takes him a long time to eat because it's hard work. But he was still able to comment on the way home, when we passed a gas station that sold fried chicken and wondered why so many gas stations sell fried chicken: "They have plenty of oil to cook it in."

We will be staying in our house at the coast for a few weeks until our Charlotte renovation is completed, with the exception of a trip to Charlotte for doctors' appointments. Come see us! Our friends have made sure the coastal house is handicap-accessible for our arrival. We expect to move back to Charlotte by mid-August. And by then, maybe Harvey won't even need what he calls "the invalid suite" for long. But it will be available for any other of our aging friends who want to visit!

This is the beginning of a different home life for us, and it will not be without challenges. Ann, who comes every weekend, is driving all the way to Charlotte on Friday just to follow us to Wilmington on Saturday in case we need her (and with two dogs, a wheelchair, walker, *cooler, suitcases, and a passenger who needs a good bit of assistance still, we certainly will). Meanwhile, we look forward to many more milestones - even the thirteens. We send our love and gratitude to each one of you and wish blessings to your families.*

CHAPTER 8

Life Goes On, Even When It Changes

We underestimate the power of a touch, a smile, a kind word, a listening ear, an honest compliment, or the smallest act of caring, all of which have the potential to turn a life around.

Leo Buscalia

Hardship and Blessings

What you learn over time about living with chronic illness is that life becomes a roller coaster. You find yourself saying repeatedly, "It's just one thing after another." Not only does progress come in fits and starts, if it comes at all, but everyday life, with its unpredictable complications, has a way of intruding. We had been excited to be going home at last. But, once again, we were writing the script as we went, and I began to resent it all.

During the weeks following the stroke, and especially when Harvey finally moved back home three months later, I became painfully aware of our dependence on others. My frequent need to inconvenience people never became comfortable, in spite of their willingness to help. Harvey and I were accustomed to being the helpers, and the role reversal from helper to the helped was one of the most difficult parts of this new life we were forced to lead. One day, when I apologized to a friend for accepting her offer of help, she said, "You know how much you guys have enjoyed helping other people over the years? Now give us the chance to help you." I remembered the enjoyment I always felt when delivering homemade soup and cookies and running errands for sick friends, mentoring and reading with children, visiting home-bound church members, and other volunteer activities. I remembered the enjoyment Harvey felt in offering legal aid and helping friends with projects. From that moment on, I vowed to be gracious and thankful rather than embarrassed and apologetic in accepting gifts of time, attention, food, and care. We could honor those gifts by helping others when we were able to do so. Meanwhile, people found many ways to assist us in our new and different life.

July 26, 2013
From: Kandy
Subject: Miracle

Sitting in the den watching the Atlanta Braves, rain dripping from the holly leaves outside the window, chocolate cake crumbs on our plates, Harvey drifting off to sleep with his legs propped up on the ottoman...this is not an unusual summer evening for us. At least, it wasn't in past summers. Everything looks so normal, from the outside. You can't see into the right side of his brain, where some of the nerve pathways are gone. You can't see all the new nerve pathways gradually forming around that black hole to compensate. You can't see the throat that couldn't swallow, the arm and leg that couldn't move, the chambers of the heart that flopped out of control. But you know it was all there. And this is what makes our good news of this week even better. Miraculous, even....

As promised, we made our great escape two weeks ago from institutional living, where improvement had happened over time. "Harvey is going home!" proclaimed the big orange poster signed by the staff: "It was a pleasure caring for you. Please come back and see us." We left the stroke blokes and animal trainers behind and headed for the coast. If Ann hadn't come from Raleigh to put Harvey in her car, I would've had to leave him there, because, with two dogs and all the stuff we had packed, I didn't have room for him in my car.

After a long, rainy trip, we unlocked the door to the house in Wilmington to find—thanks to good neighbors—flowers, balloons, food, and a house fitted with railings in all the right places. We helped Harvey to a wicker chair on the back porch while we unloaded the cars.

Not everything is going well, of course. Our insurance appeal failed for the third time. Construction in Charlotte is delayed because materials didn't arrive. The power here at the coast went out for more than twenty-four hours. Harvey's boat, the Defense Rests, began sinking in the marina because of a malfunctioning bilge pump, *whatever that is. Kind neighbors were bailing feverishly. I who know only that somehow boats are supposed to float on water was handling all the calls and sounding knowledgeable and decisive ("Just do whatever you think will work and send me the bill, and what kind of alcohol do you prefer?"), remembering that Harvey once told me "a boat is a hole in the ocean into which you pour money." Then we discovered the dishwasher was dead. Harvey's devoted sister drove an hour to stay with him so I could go out and buy the first Kitchen Aid I could find.*

Harvey can eat most foods, but all his liquids must be thickened. With a blood pressure of 80 over 48 and a heart rate of 50, he feels faint every time he stands up, often taking four or five tries over a period of ten minutes before successfully getting out of a chair. Being much lighter and shorter does not increase one's confidence in being able to help a fainting human, so at those times I am like a dogwood trying to balance a sequoia. He can never be left alone. He is exhausted. And here's the truth in all this: you can go someplace you love, but if YOU are different, then the place is not the same.

As ordered by the doctor upon Harvey's release from rehab, I have contracted with a home health agency for three types of therapists and a nurse, all of whom began calling (constantly) to schedule visits to the house. "Cosper Angels" from our neighborhood have filled our needs. They have walked our dogs, stayed with Harvey while I ran errands, performed repairs at the house, and brought groceries. One couple we have known since college drove over from Southport with two coolers full of fresh, home-prepared foods of all kinds. And gradually, things got better. Harvey has graduated from a walker to a cane. We've had to use the wheelchair just once, but we actually went to Costco together—a romantic moment for purchasing toilet paper and acid reflux reducer. We have dined out three times, with help, and Harvey didn't mind that I had to keep reminding him to wipe the left side of his mouth.

We briefly returned to Charlotte this week for two days of doctor appointments. Hearing the grandchildren talk about colossal squids and their dad's giant cannonballs into the pool gave us great joy. Harvey carefully walked up the fourteen steps to the bed that he had not seen since he was carted off, by medics, paralyzed on one side and barely able to speak, nearly one hundred days earlier. In great peace, we sat in our easy chairs and watched baseball. So now we are back at the coast for two weeks. Please come to see us, in Wilmington now, or in Charlotte in August.

And here, at last, are the miracles of this week, and of this journey:

- The feeding tube is out! Harvey passed the final swallowing test. After more than three months, he can eat and drink whatever he wants. His first thin liquid on the way home from the test at the hospital was a gigantic cup of Bojangles' sweet tea, to go with chicken and biscuits.

- The cardiologist changed medications, so that the dizziness is getting better. AND...

- Today, shadowed by the physical therapist, Harvey walked down our steps, the length of the driveway, retrieved mail from the box, and climbed back up the steps into the house...without a cane. Without assistance of any kind. Just walking! On those size thirteen feet. So this husband who has never been comfortable wearing jewelry—watch only, out of necessity—has decided to choose a small cross to wear around his neck "because I am so grateful," he says. We never for one instant have believed we deserved or earned anything that has happened to us, good or bad. But hearing from old fraternity brothers, lawyers and judges, neighbors and friends old and new, clients, friends of our children, and even strangers, so much encouragement and love, and so many miracles large and small have truly surrounded and healed us. We are God's hands and feet, and through him—through you—healing has come to our bodies and spirits.

- There is the financial advisor, a busy young father, who visited wherever we were and took on the paperwork I didn't have the time or expertise to do. There are the friends who made sure our grass was cut and the boat was safe; who hired people to install railings in our house; who stopped by with groceries and ended up staying to cook our hamburgers on the grill when Harvey tired out. The ones who rolled out our trash cans and watered plants, brought our favorite cinnamon bread, prepared goody bags for hospital sitting, took over the decorating of the new room and helped me with all the choices. Who put breakfast in my refrigerator for weeks, shared by phone late at night what it's like to care for a disabled husband, brought delicious cold suppers every Friday night for Ann and me to enjoy over the weekend. The younger lawyers (most are), secretaries, and paralegals who, on no advanced notice, took over all those cases on top of their own loads, the depositions, trials, emails, and phone calls, and managed to visit with smiles even then.

- There is the sister who stayed with Harvey for three days so I could have a break with my daughter. Those of you who sent cards or emails or who called at just those moments when I thought I couldn't do it for one more day, or one more minute. The church staff who came to pray and stayed to talk. The therapists, nurses, administrators, and aides who met every need with cheerfulness and compassion. The wooden clutching cross someone brought, the flowers, books, lunches away from the hospital. The hundreds of cards spilling loving, funny, caring thoughts into our sterile rooms like opening a window to fresh air from the ocean.

- Then there is the big, beautiful aide at Aldersgate who checked in on Harvey late one night when he was alone and very discouraged. She went up to his bed, put her arms around his head and pulled it to her chest: "Don't you worry, honey. You're gonna be all right."

> *Though we still have quite a ways to go, when you look back from April till now, everything looks so normal, from the outside. But normal is a miracle. Watching baseball together on a rainy night, sleeping in your own bed, drinking sweet tea, eating chicken and chocolate cake. Being surrounded by friends. Being with the people you love. It's all a miracle. The challenge is to remember that, and to live that way.*

For more than three months, we had wished for Harvey to be well enough to live at home for good. We knew that our daily life there would be quite different from the one we had lived together before the stroke. We knew that keeping him safe would be a constant concern, along with all the new challenges: scheduling multiple doctor and therapy appointments, helping him dress, serving foods and liquids that he could swallow without choking or aspirating, keeping up with more than thirty prescription pills to be administered at various times every day, and never being apart without arranging for someone else to stay with him. Even after more than forty years of marriage, helping my husband shower, dress, and use the bathroom felt awkward for me—my role seemed to be more that of an aide than a wife. True to his good nature, he took it all in stride with patient acceptance.

Every time Harvey stood up, he would began to sway, let out a whoosh of air, and plop back down onto the chair or bed. This would happen several times before he could finally steady himself enough to walk forward. The key was to make sure he fell back into a seat when he collapsed. Sometimes he forgot that he was not supposed to stand up or walk by himself, and he would end up on the floor. Therapists had taught us how to maneuver him back up to his knees, to leaning on a stool, to standing, but this was always difficult, especially when he was bleeding from a scrape or cut.

All this time, Harvey had little energy or interest in exercise, fresh air, or practicing what the therapists had instructed him to do. He wanted to lie down much of the time. I didn't know whether his lack of motivation was a result of the brain damage from the stroke or depression—probably both. I felt it was my job to encourage him to work at getting stronger. But it became clear that the sheer act of coming home was not going to return Harvey to the man he was before the stroke. I needed to get to know this new person and decide just how much I could expect of him. Was it helpful, or was it cruel, to continue to push him?

As it turned out, he would be fortunate just to survive the week to come.

August 18, 2013
From: Kandy
Subject: Cospers on the Rebound

Harvey Cosper is expanding his personal investigation of ambulance services and medical establishments from the Charlotte area to eastern North Carolina. A loud crash and shattering glass preceded the latest stop on the tour, this time New Hanover Regional Medical Center in Wilmington. Falling from a height of six feet four inches generally produces shock waves, though son David assures us the recent earthquakes in his city of Wellington, New Zealand, occurred several days before the Cosper incident (David's pictures fell off the walls and his six-pound dog popped up off the bed).

The tendency to faint after standing has been an impediment to Harvey's recovery. His cardiologist here is changing heart medications to elevate his heart rate and blood pressure. But this requires at least forty-eight hours of careful monitoring in the hospital to make sure it's safe and effective.

Our five weeks in Wilmington have been much busier than we expected, with in-home followed by outpatient therapy and lots of visits from friends and family. Harvey has been spotted navigating a Walmart scooter, perusing the aisles of the grocery store, cruising the Intracoastal Waterway in his own boat piloted by his brother-in-law, and actually walking out once, with help, onto the warm sands of the beach itself (he cautions that canes are no help on sand). He has enjoyed many good meals, especially fresh seafood, and a few frothy beverages, rocking on the back porch, and carefully making his way around the neighborhood's boardwalk at the edge of the water, even at night to see sunsets and falling stars. All of this activity, while exhausting, has helped him get stronger.

I recently read in Children's Letters to God:

"Dear God, how come you did all those miracles in the old days and don't do any now?

– Billy"

Life Goes On, Even When It Changes

We would love to talk to Billy and tell him miracles still do happen. Every day. A man who was paralyzed and on a feeding tube four months ago is coming home, walking and eating and talking, laughing and playing Crazy Brain games on his new iPad. He says that this experience has helped him see life more clearly—discern what's really important. This has been said so many times before that it's the king of clichés, but it's true. Someone once said that God wants spiritual fruits, not religious nuts. We certainly want to produce the former and not be the latter. But we keep thinking of Mother Teresa's famous saying: "In this life we cannot always do great things. But we can do small things with great love."

We saw this recently in the Clemson fan on the beach who noticed the trouble we were having putting up our umbrella on a windy day. It kept blowing onto his encampment of tents, chairs, surfboards and coolers clearly meant for a family with kids. In spite of Harvey's Carolina tee shirt, this stranger in his orange paw-printed cap took over the project for us and made it work using a sandbag. Later, as we were packing up to leave, having learned a little about us from my sister, the young father walked back over and knelt in front of Harvey's chair. "Sir, I just wanted to wish you a good recovery. Would it be all right if I prayed for you?" And right there on the beach, we took off our caps and, in a circle, bowed our heads as he prayed for Harvey's continued healing. (NOTE: I sent this story to the Charlotte Observer *for their "Everyday*

> Angels" series, and it was published that September.)
>
> Even though our renovation isn't quite finished, we plan to be back in Charlotte this Saturday for at least a month—assuming Harvey gets out of the hospital in a couple of days and the heart medications are working well. We've installed a ramp and shower bars, and he should be able to manage the stairs carefully for now. We appreciate our church's setting up a website for meals and a care team of guys for visiting Harvey. Please call and come see us! We want to hear what's happening in your lives.
>
> Meanwhile, we will be happy to share our extensive—almost all positive—evaluations of hospitals, ambulance services, rehab facilities, doctors, handicap equipment, home up-fitting outfits, and insurance plans with you, even as we pray you won't have to deal with any of them yourself. Most of all, we can share so many stories of kindness, thoughtfulness, caring, and concern, stories of angels sent to us by a loving God. Really.

Although my emails to our friends percolated with positive and grateful vibes, I had come to terms with the possibility—no, the fact—that life would never be the same for us. Assuring my husband's safety required constant vigilance. At no time was this clearer than when I found Harvey sprawled on our back porch steps, bleeding from the head, unconscious, and no longer breathing.

A Near-Death Experience

Following a three-day stint in the hospital after the latest fall, we had been back at our Wilmington house for just three hours before Harvey nearly lost his life. He and I were sitting on the back porch in the afternoon sun, sipping iced tea (well, his glass held tea), looking past the wide gray steps to the small patch of green grass and the yellow flowers along the fence. Fresh summer vegetables simmered on the stove. Leaving the back door open, I had just stepped inside to check on dinner when I heard a thud. I could see out the window that Harvey's chair was empty.

I found him lying face down, unmoving, with his feet on the porch and his head on a lower step, blood spreading into the wood. He did not appear to be breathing. I called 911 and, phone in hand, ran next door.

Once again, a coincidence that I considered a miracle occurred: our next-door-neighbors' daughter and her husband happened to be having a rare weeknight dinner there, and they are both doctors of chiropractic. They ran through the gate to Harvey's still form and, as I hovered over them murmuring "Oh God, oh God," they went to work. They turned him over. A deep blue color was rising in his face like water filling a vase, and they could not find a pulse. Immediately, the young man began chest compressions. Within less than a minute, as sirens wailed closer, Harvey made a gurgling noise. An ambulance and two fire trucks arrived, spilling out a horde of helpful people.

For the first time in a lifetime of being asked, Harvey didn't know who he was or where he was. But slowly, as they loaded him onto a stretcher, he began to speak. As the medics departed, the neighbors and fire fighters were hosing down the steps.

A well-known professor of religion at UNC, Dr. Bernard Boyd, used to teach us that a miracle is not necessarily what happens, but that it happens at the right time. Scientists can try to explain away the ten plagues of Moses, the turning of water into wine, or the rolling away of Jesus' gravestone, he told us, but it's the timing of those events that shows God's intent. I don't want to think about what would have happened had our doctor friends not been visiting at that time.

Harvey never regained any memory of the events of that evening. He asked me repeatedly what happened, whether we were in a wreck, where he was found. Did he try to stand up? Did he have a seizure and then fall? We will never know. He certainly looked as if he has been in a wreck. His face was swollen to the point of being unrecognizable, the skin was stripped from his arms, and he was sore from head to toe. But X-rays and CT scans revealed not one inner bleed, not one broken bone.

We spent a grueling eight-hour night in the Emergency Department before moving to Cardiac Intensive Care. As I left for home the next morning to check on the dogs, shower, and once again collect some of his belongings, Harvey asked me to pick up a suit of armor for him or, at the very least, a sturdy football helmet.

Sometime later, when he next saw the doctors who had saved his life, he looked at the lovely young woman and said, "I hope you were the one who gave me mouth-to-mouth."

Life Goes On, Even When It Changes

August 13, 2013
Ann's Facebook Post

Dad's spent the past week at the hospital due to a bad fall. Please don't contact Mom right now as she has a lot on her plate, but feel free to leave well-wishes on here. We expect Dad to be out of the hospital in the next few days, followed by a few days in rehab in Charlotte and then hopefully home.

#dadquote

- "Pain is inevitable. It's like frying bacon in the nude. You know it's gonna hurt, you just don't know when or where."
- On hospital meals: "The puréed chicken looked like dog poop and the puréed green beans looked like goose poop."
- On his post-fall appearance: "I look like I've been through a meat grinder."
- On his compression socks: "All I'm missing is a garter belt."

Thanks for your continued support and prayers for him and my incredible, resilient, tireless, devoted mom.

BTW: There are two Department of Corrections officers in bulletproof vests with our next door neighbor here at all times. Keeps things exciting.

A Warning about Health Insurance

I never calculated the cumulative cost of Harvey's medical care but, by this point, four months post-stroke, I estimate the bills totaled close to a million dollars. We paid into an employee health insurance plan that had covered nearly every necessary expense. Unfortunately, when Harvey turned sixty-five that summer, I failed to do the right thing.

A person turning sixty-five is automatically enrolled in Medicare A for hospital expenses. There is a prescribed window of time in which to enroll in Part B for medical expenses. The health insurance coverage year through Harvey's firm ran from September first to August thirty-first and, at his sixty-fifth birthday in June, two months after the stroke, I saw no reason to change. A professional insurance advisor agreed. Harvey was on short-term disability at the time, and we still hoped he would eventually return to work. So I elected to stay with the employee plan and did not sign him up for Medicare B. This turned out to be one of the most expensive decisions I ever made.

In late summer, we received notification that the law firm was switching health plan carriers as of September first, so I visited the Social Security office to enroll Harvey in Medicare B. The representative told me I should have known that, if you don't sign up for Medicare during the grace period around your birthday, when you do enroll, you have a two-month waiting period: the earliest Harvey could start with Medicare B would be November first. So I enrolled Harvey in the new "full coverage" employee plan at a high premium for the two months before Medicare B took effect.

Life Goes On, Even When It Changes

What I didn't know was that, once you are eligible for Medicare, whether or not you actually enroll, private insurance policies generally are just supplemental: they cover only twenty percent of medical expenses. Unfortunately, in those next two months, Harvey had serious medical emergencies that required more hospitalizations and rehab.

In the ensuing months, huge medical bills began to arrive in our mailbox. *These are just copies,* I thought; *we don't really owe all this; the interim insurance policy will cover it all.* I was so busy going to and from the hospital, taking care of Harvey and dealing with one crisis after another, that it took me a few weeks to realize what was going on: most of Harvey's medical bills were no longer being paid by insurance. A few phone calls and apologetic emails later, the bad news sank in: insurance was covering at most twenty percent of the bills, and they totaled more than three hundred thousand dollars.

Eventually, the law firm assigned us an independent benefits advisor. Though we never met in person, "Mary from Winston-Salem" was professional and caring. I faxed her more than sixty pages of unpaid medical bills which she worked through, sending the hospital portions to Medicare A and renegotiating the medical amounts from their original premium retail rates. It took many months and many phone calls and lots of paperwork, but the total we owed was reduced considerably. Still, I was forced to spend much of Harvey's disability income and savings to cover those expenses. Once again, his long-ago decision to purchase disability coverage kept us from having to sell assets we had intended to support us during retirement.

Thirteenth Relocation

During our weeks in Wilmington, we had been living fairly peacefully, leaving the house several times a week for shopping, eating at restaurants, and driving to outpatient rehab. Harvey was working on cognitive issues such as focusing, left side neglect, puzzle solving, and reading, as well as the physical ones. He was doing more things for himself, even cooking breakfast for us. He walked slowly with a cane. We were keeping the Sweet's Syndrome episodes fairly well under control with medication. I had gotten used to administering the meds, wrapping wounds, preparing the shower and a big dry towel afterwards, pulling on socks and buttoning his shirts. We were sleeping beside each other once again. Still, I had not been able to keep him safe.

The small fall and the great fall, followed by eleven more days in the hospital, were major setbacks. For weeks his face was so many colorful shades that he claimed to be "a glow-in-the-dark dad" for his kids: "I look like the wreck of the Hesperus." His painful arms, which had lost much of their skin, were wrapped like a mummy's. For a while, he had even been put back on thickened liquids and soft foods—tough for a person who finally got rid of a feeding tube.

When it came time to leave the hospital, once again he was not allowed to go directly home. As before, he was prescribed the intermediate step of more inpatient rehabilitation. We decided on a smaller Charlotte hospital he had yet to try. With sadness and disappointment, I packed up our suitcases from Wilmington, filled a cooler with leftovers, loaded the two dogs in the back of the car, and picked up Harvey in front of the hospital for the four-hour drive back. He was carsick the entire trip and, when we pulled up to the front of the rehab hospital, he threw up at the curb all over himself and an aide who had come forward with a wheelchair.

Oh, no, I thought—*here we go again. Back to a place of sickness. Back to hospital beds, wheelchairs, call buttons, and boredom. Back to living apart.*

As it turned out, Harvey made little progress in rehab this time. The "drop attacks," as he called them, limited the therapists' ability to work with him. He began having what appeared to be seizures, most often when he was laid back too quickly in bed. I could not help out as much, because his room was so tiny that I had to step out every time a nurse or aide entered—which was often. Once again, the prospect of coming home—this time, finally, in Charlotte—loomed, for both of us, as both happy and frightening. How in the world would we manage?

September 8, 2013
From: Kandy
Subject: Harvey is coming home this week

In the 148 days since his stroke in April, Harvey Cosper has spent 109 days in seven different medical institutions, been rushed by ambulance to four emergency rooms, suffered through five hospitalizations, participated in five inpatient rehabilitation programs and been relocated a total of twelve times. The thirteenth relocation will be this Thursday, when he can finally return to our

Charlotte home. *This continues the run of (un)lucky thirteens I mentioned in an earlier update: born on June thirteenth, stroke on April thirteenth in 2013, released from rehab to home on July thirteenth after exactly thirteen weeks—and, believe it or not, his last ER room in Wilmington was number thirteen and his room number on the floor ended in thirteen. This week, his first full day at home in Charlotte will be Friday the thirteenth and he will be wearing his size thirteen sneakers.*

Harvey's luck has seemed to run out repeatedly this year. This latest rehab stint has been a terribly disappointing step backward to wheelchairs, walkers, bed and chair alarms, and very little walking or self-care. Because he gets dizzy much of the time upon changing position, and because his falls have been life-threatening, the staff has been understandably cautious.

Even so, they had to call a Code Blue for a blackout last week. It's scary to see medical people running from all directions to crowd around your loved one, who is sprawled on the floor, with their gadgets and machines and shouting orders to one another. Since the stroke, at least four cardiologists, three neurologists, and several other specialists have performed countless tests and adjusted his medications many times. His vital signs are checked multiple times each day. To increase blood pressure and stability, his legs and mid-section are wrapped tightly before he is allowed into physical therapy. Still, no one has a definitive solution to the problem. A pacemaker is

Life Goes On, Even When It Changes

being considered, but some of the doctors don't feel it will help much. All this has greatly interfered with his ability to work at the rehabilitation he must have—especially in these critical first six months following a stroke when optimal improvements can be made.

He will be released this week to "24/7 supervision," meaning I will not be able to leave him alone until and unless the blackout problem is solved. There will be more weeks of in-home and outpatient rehab, depending upon insurance. We continued to have trouble with insurance coverage. When I was complaining about having to make more of the countless calls and visits to those entities, Harvey suggested I just go online to www.weain'tpayin.com or call 1-800-kissmyass. The care team organized by our parish nurse will be very helpful, as will the scheduled meals. Somehow, I will find a way to resume some of my own outside activities, and somehow it will all work out over time.

Meanwhile, I can't deny that we have had some really long, hard days —hard times emotionally as well as physically; days when it's been hard to smile and not to weep. Days when it seems we have taken two steps forward only to take two steps back. I hope that we can finally stop counting days in institutions and start counting beautiful fall days at home, time with our family and friends, days when no one falls or stops breathing, no one gets medications mixed up, no one asks me where I want to put light switches or when I will have the latest forms filled out.

From the beginning of this journey, the bad luck has been balanced by the blessings along the way—especially the expressions of love and concern from so many people. The angels just keep on visiting us. Thanks to the help of dear friends, I was able to fly back to Wilmington for the funeral last week of a close friend and pastor. His memorial service was sad but inspiring, as he had helped to make life better for so many people. We were reminded to think about what we want written on our tombstones, as a way of determining how we want to live our lives, and to think about how our lives touch others. Countless people have touched us in many ways, helping us through the bad times and leaving us with hope. And so it's impossible to feel victimized by "bad luck," even in our lowest moments. We can't help but see the face of God and feel the hand of God every day in the people who care for us. Today after a church service at the hospital, among other physically and mentally damaged people, Harvey said he was reminded of the constant presence of God, a presence he never forgets.

A sign beside Harvey's hospital room door last week quoted Joseph Addison in words often repeated by football coach Lou Holtz: "Four grand essentials to happiness in this life are something to do, something to love, something to believe in, and something to hope for." We have all of these. And we hope you do, too. Please come see us when you can. It will be so good to be home!

Life Goes On, Even When It Changes

September 14, 2013
Ann's Facebook Post

Dad came home from his latest hospital/rehab stint on Thursday. Today we bought him some new clothes for his new, slight frame, which were still too big, but he wore them anyway to our first nice dinner out in six months. Dad's different, but there he was, all cleaned up and wearing the kind of clothing I've known him to wear for the past twenty-nine years. Kandy Cosper looked stunning as usual, and we headed downtown to celebrate a new start.

We saw (basketball legend) Patrick Ewing at dinner, but that may have been the least important part of the evening. We have never been treated so specially as we were tonight. My friend, the restaurant manager, saw to it that our first nice meal back in the real world was one for the record books. We enjoyed bread and butter, wine, tenderloin skewers, lobster bisque, chopped salads, flawlessly cooked filets, lobster, stuffed chicken, a crab cake, potatoes au gratin, asparagus with hollandaise, creamed spinach, chocolate lava cake with vanilla ice cream, and coffee. And I may be forgetting something. Everything we could have wanted was taken care of before we knew we wanted it. My friend even had the executive chef himself come out, and he cut my dad's entree into manageable, bite-sized pieces.

We were treated tonight with the utmost care and service, but in a different way than we have been used to *for the past months. Tonight, we were treated like adult human beings with dignity. My dad was more cheerful tonight than he has been since his stroke. Exhausted and grateful, we returned to my parents' beautiful home where I grew up, got into our pajamas, and sat on the back porch on this beautiful night, enjoying the sounds of the cicadas and crickets and each other's laughter until we all began to doze off.*

I think when David in Psalm 23 says, "My cup runneth over," this is what he's talking about. With a full belly and an even fuller heart, I'm not sure I've ever been more grateful for all my blessings than I am right now.

CHAPTER 9

WHEN HOME IS NOT THE SAME, EPISODE 2

Faith is not about everything turning out okay. It's about being okay no matter how things turn out.

author unknown

So we were finally home in Charlotte, greeted by crisp fall weather, family, friends, a poster signed by the neighbors, good food, and a convenient new space. Harvey restarted outpatient rehabilitation. The first photo I shared in the group email since our ordeal began was of Harvey, Ann, and me together at church for the first time in months. His face was shades of black, yellow, and blue, and he had a big white bandage above one eye. He must have looked ten years older to the people who had last seen him months earlier, before the stroke. But, after being on the congregational prayer list for almost half a year, he was finally sitting in the pew, and we felt loved and celebrated by so many who had prayed for us for many months.

Being home together was good. Harvey could climb the stairs to our bedroom at night, and he used the new downstairs room for daytime rest. Although scheduling was a logistical puzzle involving untold phone calls and constant changes, therapists were coming to the house to help with walking, dressing, and other everyday activities as well as exercises. Eventually, we would drive to therapy and, finally, to a private trainer at our church gym. I began to think of outside activities Harvey might enjoy, since his chief interests of working and boating were not feasible for him.

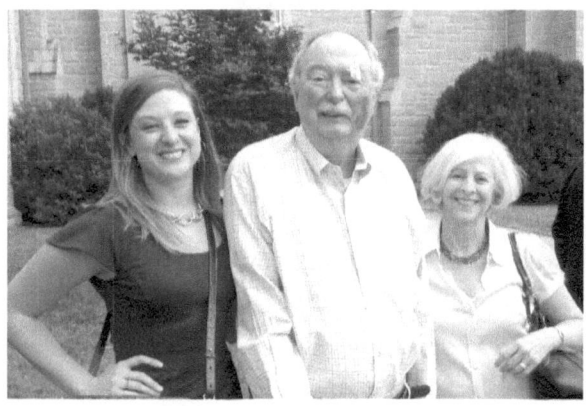

Harvey's first Sunday back at church, five months after the stroke and five weeks after the Big Fall, with daughter and wife

But, once again, being home was also hard for both of us. I was surprised that Harvey did not seem more excited to be there. I didn't know whether his stroke had so changed his ability to express emotions such as excitement and joy, or whether he was unable even to feel those emotions. When I asked him, he responded, "Probably both."

The truth is that home is not the same when you are not the same. He wanted to go back to work. He wanted to be useful.

When Home is Not the Same, Episode 2

He wanted to walk on the beach and play ball with the grandchildren. He grieved for the daily life he had lost. His sense of humor never failed—the one-liners kept coming. His beautiful prayers at mealtimes were a testament to his strong faith. But he was exhausted, physically and emotionally, and he wanted to rest most of the time. He lost interest in being outdoors. He seemed to feel he was on the fringes of life. One especially poignant afternoon, he sat quietly on the porch watching the grandchildren and me playing whiffle ball in the yard. He later commented, "I will never be able to play with them like that again. They will remember me as a sick old man."

As it turned out, Harvey was home for only a matter of days before being rushed to the hospital following another bad fall. And there were many falls after that. We began making friends with the first responders from the local fire department. I learned to tell the 911 operator that I needed just "lift assist" when there wasn't much blood, so the sirens did not blare through the streets and bring the neighbors running outside in alarm. These kind men and women never seemed to mind coming. Harvey always had something funny to say to them, even when he was lying on the floor amid splatters of red.

Just keeping a list of all the medical providers and medications was a big job, and I caused myself many problems by not having been organized enough in preceding years. Once again, caring people came to the rescue. Our financial advisor visited us regularly to help us decide how to deal with medical bills, insurance, and disability income, and make plans for the future. We included Harvey in some of the discussions, but he was unable to concentrate on the details. Gradually, I made my way through the morass of paperwork, reminding doctors' office staff to fill out disability forms and letters of appeal.

Harvey coped with his many challenges by not taking himself too seriously and not feeling sorry for himself. He continued to express gratitude. We tried to be honest and open with ourselves and others. We read aloud, listened to music, and tackled word puzzles together. But the greatest blessing of all was our caring friends and family.

Practical Help for Sick Friends at Home

Never let your quest for perfection frustrate your ability to do good.

Harvey Cosper, Jr.,
quoting a source he couldn't remember

Once we were back home, the pent-up desire of friends who wanted to help but could not during the incarcerations burst forth in ways we never could have imagined. Several nights a week, a cooler on our front steps filled with delicious meals. This is one of the best gifts we can give people living at home with chronic illness: **provide meals, delivering them in disposable containers that do not have to be washed and returned.**

Friends and congregations can **organize to provide ongoing support.** A care team of folks signed up to stay with Harvey on

Thursday nights so that I could attend choir practice. Harvey enjoyed their visits, and what a joy it was for me to be singing again among my friends of so many years. The care team also served as a convenient list to call when we needed extra visits or, as he called it, "babysitting" at other times. He most appreciated **visitors who are relaxed and do not demand too much interaction.** They brought books and could sit quietly if he felt tired. They watched sporting events on TV and did not ask too many questions. Conversation flowed gently and easily.

After Harvey's stroke, one of the biggest surprises was the people who visited regularly. Again, some of the people who visited most faithfully were folks we had known only casually. We enjoyed these newer friendships, the interesting conversation, the news of the outside world and of their families.

As illness stretched into disability over many months, we heard from fewer friends and colleagues. This is to be expected; people have their own routines and busy lives. We had done the same in the past—visited sick friends at the time of crisis and then had little contact later. But, in a way, we cherished connection with others even more in this phase of chronic illness than in those first weeks after the stroke. People who **continue to pay attention to the family over the long months** truly help to keep the spirits up.

I especially appreciated **acts of kindness and helpfulness to the children.** Other members of the family were having a tough time, too. When our daughter had a good friend bring her a meal, send her a card, or offer to care for her dog, or when our sons had friends ask about and acknowledge the difficulties of having a dad who was sick, this meant so much to all of us.

In addition to the helpful actions included in my earlier list, here are some practical things that people said and did for us during those first weeks at home. Many are similar to the favors people had been offering us since the stroke, and they made life easier for us.

- "Let me come and visit with Harvey for a couple of hours so you can get out."
- Texting before dropping by for short visits (less than 30 minutes).
- Rolling the garbage cans out and back on trash day without being asked.
- "I am taking Harvey's car for a wash. When will it need an inspection?"
- "I'll take care of it. You have enough to think about."
- Participating in online signup for food and care teams.
- Bringing food frozen in small quantities.
- Ironing clothes.
- Planting, sweeping the porch, picking up sticks and branches in the yard.
- Sending flowers and cards.
- Picking a night to offer a choice of dinner: eat at our house or yours together, or drop off food.
- Offering restaurant takeout.
- "What do you need at (Target, post office, pharmacy)? I'm going shopping tomorrow."
- "Is there a doctor appointment for which I can help with transportation?"

- "I like to…" (cook, update technology, shop, do yard work, iron, etc.); when can I do this for you?"
- In conversation, forgiving me when I was tired and insensitive.
- Reflecting our feelings and circumstances: "I'm so happy you feel good about your medical team." "I'm so glad your children could be here." "So many people care about you."
- When we apologized for being a burden, being gracious with us. One person actually said, "It's a privilege."

In addition to the care teams, we appreciated our church's intercessory prayer team and the live-streaming of our services for online worship when we could not get there in person. On the screen, we saw our friends in the pews and we heard Harvey's name as they prayed for him. If he was in the hospital or in rehab, the nurses would stop in to watch the service. Home visits by church staff and home communion were very meaningful. We also received cards and notes regularly on behalf of the congregation.

In summary, the most important suggestion I have for people who wish to help is this: **stay connected. Continue to let the family know you are thinking of them during the tedious, challenging months when home is not the same anymore.**

As I look back, what I appreciate most is the people who came—the ones who showed up—offering **the ministry of presence.** This is the best gift of all.

Repeating Ourselves

September 21, 2013
From: Kandy
Subject: Harvey is acting up again

Harvey has been admitted to the hospital—again—following two medic visits for falling today. A pacemaker is being discussed, but they don't think it will necessarily solve the problem. His arm infections will have to be dealt with first. He is currently scarfing down a cheeseburger. This is the eighth medical emergency admission since April, but we continue to hope for the best.

September 26, 2013
From: Kandy
Subject: He's Got Rhythm

This fall day could not be more beautiful out here on the porch. The only problem is that Harvey, once again, is not here to enjoy it with me. This time he was home eight days before three more falls—two requiring ambulance and medics—finally put him back in Carolinas Medical Center. We have lost count of the total number of hospitalizations and are now counting lost seasons...spring, summer, now a few days of...wait, Ann says we have to eliminate the term "fall" and call it "autumn" instead.

The hopeful news is that yesterday a pacemaker was installed in his chest. The cardiologists tell us that this little disk, with its two thin wires corkscrewed into the

When Home is Not the Same, Episode 2

heart, will not solve all his problems, but they think it could help.

The week at home in between hospitalizations was "the best of times and the worst of times," as Dickens would say. We enjoyed the kindness and presence of many good friends, started outpatient rehab (again), ate some wonderful meals, slept in our own bed, and marveled at the simple pleasures of living at home, with its old and new spaces. Although one night Harvey woke up thrashing around in the bed and, when I asked what the matter was, he told me he was looking for the call button to ring the nurse. I told him the nurse was sleeping in the bed with him.

However, Harvey could never be left even in a room by himself. He was too emotionally and physically exhausted to work much at recouping all his losses. The scheduling of appointments and sitters became overwhelming, and I missed simple things like walking my dogs and going to Curves in the mornings. The magnitude of the changes in our life together covered us like a gray fog.

Last Saturday, I was attending the funeral of a friend, then headed to an afternoon retreat with the Covenant choir, when sweet Ann's voicemail message came in: "Dad fell twice and the medics are here. Don't worry and please don't come home." Then a text message: "Going to the hospital just to make sure he doesn't have a brain bleed. Go ahead to your activities," followed by "We are in the ER, room 8" (not 13 this time!). I responded from my spot at the church under a tree dripping with rain: "Locked keys in car. Friend on way with second set. Will come as soon as I can."

Meanwhile, the veteran hospital patient has maintained his usual aplomb. When someone asked him his name, he responded, "My name is Lazarus." When asked if he still felt as though a truck had run over him, he said, "I think he backed up and ran over me again." After his latest EEG, he told us that "there were strobe lights in there. They should have been playing Jimi Hendrix." And he told a nurse who recognized him from a previous admission, "I've got to stop hanging out in places like this."

Yesterday morning I saw a rainbow arching across the sky. Our church's small group Bible study of Genesis had just reached the story of Noah and the rainbow that sealed God's covenant to continue saving and caring for the human race. It is a symbol both of continuing and of starting over. We know that we are under that divine care and, when Harvey leaves the hospital tomorrow, we will be simultaneously continuing and starting over. The pacemaker will not help his low blood pressure, but it will keep Harvey's heart rate in a reasonable range. It will also allow the doctors to add stronger medications to keep him out of atrial fibrillation. Harvey is very weak, but he has regained his determination to work hard at getting better.

I have been trying to keep up with everything but have shown a few understandable signs of mental crack-up. I have missed a few bills—including quarterly taxes—and still haven't written to thank the many people who continue to help us in every way. Sunday evening I came home from the hospital tired and frustrated, with calls to return, but my cell phone was dead. So I plugged it into the wall and picked up the house phone to call Ann, who had just driven back to Raleigh. No sooner had I dialed than my cell phone began to ring again. In disgust, I barked "HELLO!" and - it was me. I had called myself. When I redialed to reach Ann, she said with her usual dry wit, "Well, I hope you at least had a good conversation." I replied, "No, I hung up on myself."

But we have a lot to look forward to. David is coming home just before Halloween for nearly two weeks—for the first time since the weeks following the stroke in April! Harvey's sister and her son are coming to visit from Texas for the first time in years. The grandchildren will make sure the Force is with us in their Star Wars costumes for Halloween. Lots of good meals and good friends are showing up at our house. Rehab appointments stretch through the fall. And my sister and her husband have invited Harvey for a fun weekend in horse country around Durham so that I can relax among fall leaves taking in dear friends' spectacular views in the NC mountains in October. We trust all these things will happen, and all ambulances and hospital beds will be avoided.

Once again, I am hoping this is the last Cosper email you will have to receive. We don't count on that anymore, however. Not much is for sure in this life. But I have carried with me the program from Saturday's "Witness *to the Resurrection Celebrating the Life" of a brave and cheerful younger friend who suffered long from cancer. It reads, from Isaiah, "...Those who wait for the Lord shall renew their strength, they shall mount up with wings like eagles, they shall run and not be weary, they shall walk and not faint."*

We are especially excited about the walking and not fainting part.

With love and appreciation to each of you.

October 3, 2013
Ann's Facebook Post

Dad has been in the hospital for a couple of weeks due to his inability to stand and/or walk without getting dizzy and falling and hurting himself and/or others. Of course, being in a hospital bed for weeks has further deconditioned him. He will be at CMC through Monday, at which time we'll have to decide what's next. Doctors are grasping at straws at this point trying to make things better. I'd be lying if I didn't say morale is low. I will be back in Charlotte at the hospital this weekend, if anyone wants to stop by and say hello to us.

October 4, 2013
From: Kandy
Subject: Short report on long, hard times

I seem to be repeating myself with these emails, because the same things keep happening. Harvey is still

When Home is Not the Same, Episode 2

in the hospital, two weeks after falling at home. Thanks to the new pacemaker, his heart is working well. His infected arms are healing. But, as the doctors warned, he continues to have fainting spells and seizure-like episodes, and the list of possible diagnoses is getting shorter. Meanwhile, Harvey is completing his eighteenth week in a medical institution out of the past twenty-five weeks.

Although he could have been released from the cardiac floor (the best nursing experience we have ever had), and we join him in wanting so badly for him to come home, we know it's not safe right now. We are considering our options, including some additional rehab. He is starting two new medications this weekend, and he will be released on Monday to have more tests away from the hospital. At least there is a lot of good baseball to watch, and the broadcasts happen to be on one of the few hospital channels. And, since they didn't play last weekend, the Panthers did not lose.

It's hard for him to remain hopeful after so many setbacks. It's hard for me to see his car in the driveway covered with dust and leaves, his red cap on the dresser, and his empty chair when I come home alone after a long day.

We do look forward to better days. Just maybe my next email will be the last—telling you that the problems are solved and we are home together for good. We appreciate your prayers for our strength, gratitude, and patience as we work through these difficult times.

CHAPTER 10

WHEN A NEW NORMAL NEVER COMES

Caregiving often calls us to lean into love we didn't know possible.
Tia Walker, *The Inspired Caregiver: Finding Joy While Caring for Those You Love*

In October, six months after the stroke, following another long hospitalization, Harvey was sent back to the rehabilitation building for another, shorter stint. This time, he knew what to expect: three hours a day of hard work, the rest of the time spent in bed.

Meanwhile, a new problem was worsening: being laid flat on a bed or exercise table precipitated a seizure. His eyes would roll back, his left arm and leg would curl inward and, for about ten seconds, he would be unresponsive. When he came to, he couldn't remember what had happened.

The nurses, therapists, and I had observed this a number of times, but the doctors never had. So the therapists invited two of the physicians on staff to come to the therapy room to see if they could induce an episode. Several times they had Harvey sit on the edge of the therapy table before quickly laying him flat, and several times the frightening seizures occurred.

Harvey had had a number of scans and MRIs of his head—from the night of the stroke to the hospitalizations for his falls, faints, and seizures. This time, the neurologists scheduled him for an EEG to detect abnormal activity. While he was sitting up, they covered his balding head with multi-colored electrodes; he looked like an alien from a comedic old horror movie. Suddenly, a technician lowered the back of the bed; Harvey remained calm and conscious. The test was repeated several times, but, unlike the experiment in the therapy room, this one did not cause any adverse reactions: they could not make it happen when they most needed to. It reminded me of calling AAA when your car won't start, only to have it start right up when they arrive. The doctors prescribed seizure medication, anyway, in case it would help.

After the brain tests, we made even more signs to go over his bed along with the signs advising no tape on his skin. These read: "Do Not Lay Flat." More than once, aides who missed the memo were frightened as the patient floundered for several seconds before regaining consciousness. This was just one more problem that interfered with his ability to exercise and participate fully in physical and occupational therapy.

During this time, someone ran into my car in the hospital parking lot, causing several thousand dollars in damage. No note was left. After notifying the insurance company, I had to take the car to the dealership for a repair estimate, solicit rides to and from the service department, and transfer to Harvey's car, which needed to be driven, anyway. Inconveniences like this—

not pleasurable in the best of times—are especially trying during stressful times of illness, although damage to a car seemed so much less important than ever before. Even though I suspected Harvey would never drive that car again, keeping it seemed to be a sign of hope for him, whereas selling it would have been a sign of giving up.

Meanwhile, when Harvey's sister and nephew made a rare visit from Texas, all four of his siblings and two of the three step-siblings enjoyed time together on the patio of the rehab hospital. We have pictures of them smiling, surrounding their oldest brother as he sat in a wheelchair in shorts and a tee shirt, his face, arms, and legs splotched with bruises and bandages. It would be the last time they would all get together.

One Page from the Spouse's Notebook

As I look back at my stack of small frayed, stained notebooks from those first six months, my name and address sticker on the front smudged and torn, I discover a timeline that sums up Harvey's journey to this point. In various pens and pencils, words curl around the margins and run off the edges.

Front:
    4/7 – Hospital – a-fib and Sweet's
    4/10 – home
    4/13 – stroke. Hospital. Neuro ICU. Cardiac ICU
    4/13 - regular room

4/29 –Carolinas Rehab
5/23 – Home
5/27 – Asbury Nursing Home
6/13 – Hospital
6/19 – Asbury
7/13 – Wilmington house
7/22-25 – Charlotte, doctors
7/25 – 8/17 – Wilmington house
8/17- Hospital
8/18- Home
8/18-8/28 –Wilmington hospital
8/28-9/12 – Wilmington house
9/12-9/21 – Home to Charlotte
9/21-10/8- Hospital
10/8-10/24 – Inpatient rehab in Charlotte

BACK:
Random notes including contact names, a handicap-equipment dealer, insurance information, a quotation from a wall at the hospital, reminders, grocery items, and an anonymous telephone number.

After this, the notebooks continued, but I gave up on keeping a timeline.

November 9, 2013
From: Kandy
Subject: For all the saints
  Last Sunday, assisted by Ann, Harvey Cosper joined

the procession of worshippers making their way up the aisle of the beautiful sanctuary of Covenant Presbyterian Church. One at a time, he carefully selected tall white spider mums and placed them reverently into a vase in memory of a friend and of our parents, all of whom have preceded us into the next life. It was All Saints Day and, from my perch in the choir, I saw many eyes being wiped as the bell rang in remembrance of people we have loved and no longer see on this earth. It was one of the few Sundays in the past seven months that Harvey's name was not on the hospital or prayer list in the bulletin. I wept to see my frail husband so typically remembering other people when he himself had lost so much that year. But he does not see life in terms of losses; he sees it in terms of blessings, and he knows that he has much to be thankful for. We sang "For All the Saints" and, being diehard Presbyterians, we count many living saints among our friends in "the priesthood of all believers."

I will confess that I counseled him not to go forward during the evening service of the choir's "Requiem" to light candles in memory of people, even though David was safely with him, as we would be sad to burn down such a lovely church.

We have been home more than two weeks now without a fall or a hospitalization. This is good news! Harvey says he was "released from prison" in time for David's trip home from New Zealand. We celebrated Thanksgiving as a complete family for the first time in five years—three weeks early—and Harvey helped with the turkey and dressing, as always.

He has four to six hours of outpatient therapy per week. We have appointments at wound care, doctors' offices, and labs every week. We have a fine fellow coming to the house three mornings a week to help get the day started, which gives me a chance to exercise and get some errands done.

Harvey is gentle and sweet to care for, but I tend to have too much energy and not enough patience for the job. Never has the corny old saying "one day at a time" been more appropriate for us than it has been this year.

Although he needs to rest a lot, Harvey has been seen voting at the polls, eating a hot dog on East Blvd., grocery shopping, walking down the driveway, and giving out Halloween candy on Graham and Lisa's front porch while our little Anakin Skywalker and Padmé Amidala collected candy around the block. We even got our picture taken for the church directory in celebration of the fact that, as Harvey says, he is "still fogging the glass." He has lost so much hair since the last picture, and the right side of his face sags, but then I'm not one to talk—both sides of my face are sagging. Upon seeing himself on the proofs on a computer screen, he exclaimed, "Who is that old goat?" He was happy to answer a call or two from the office on legal matters. Anyone willing to come help him adjust to his iPhone and iPad, please don't hang back from volunteering.

This morning we were eating pancakes and remembering how much Harvey dreamed about them when he was being fed through a tube. We started to compare the food at the all the hospitals and rehabs until we got disgusted and talked about sports instead—miraculously, our teams are all winning this week. We continue to dream of taking a real vacation, maybe a river cruise, and each boring exercise and mouthful of medication is a step in that direction.

We hope to get out Thanksgiving cards. Whether we do or not, please consider yourself thanked for reading our messages and for being our friends. So many saints we are blessed to know! A joyous Thanksgiving to everyone.

December 19, 2013
Ann's Facebook Post

When Khloe [Kardashian] and Lamar announced that they were divorcing, I thought love was over. But I'm reminded today, on my parents' forty-third anniversary, that love hasn't gone anywhere, and that real love never gives up. My mom and dad have been through "for better or worse." They have been through "for richer or poorer." This year was all about "in sickness and in health."

Kandy Cosper had just transferred from Randolph-Macon to UNC-Chapel Hill when she met Dad on a blind date. He became her rock, and she became his sparkle. She became the sweetheart of his fraternity. They were twenty-two and broke and fresh out of college when they got married in 1970. Dad had just gotten out of the army. Mom never had an engagement ring, and she wore *her cousin's dress on her wedding day. Of course, no one remembered to pick up Dad on the day of the wedding. Her grandfather called the church to remind them, someone rushed out, and there he was, in his tux, smoking a cigarette on the curb waiting for his ride. They had a humble noon ceremony at First Presbyterian Church in Greensboro, followed by a covered dish luncheon, cookies and punch, and a receiving line at the church. For their honeymoon, they spent two nights in Williamsburg, Virginia.*

Mom worked at an insurance company and put Dad through Wake Forest law school. She gave birth to Graham on April 28, 1975, during my dad's final law school exams. He studied for the bar exam with a newborn baby in the room and sometimes in his lap. Dad had one job offer, and he took it. They moved to Charlotte. Then came David, and then, much later, surprise! there I was. (Dad always says it's a good thing I came last, because they wouldn't have been able to afford me any earlier.)

It's always annoyed Mom that Dad picks up his salad bowl at dinner. It annoys Dad that Mom nags him about various things. She is five-feet-three and he is six-feet-four. She is loud and he is quiet. She is excitable and he is calm. In a lot of ways, they are quite opposite. But they have the important things in common, which is why they are still together. And he can always, always make her laugh.

At this point, nagging and picking up salad bowls are the farthest things from their minds. Sitting in some hospital room at some point this year, I saw my mom gingerly navigate all of Dad's IVs and feeding tube and crawl into his hospital bed. She lay down next to him, and she helped him put his bad arm around her, and they lay there and watched the Atlanta Braves together, talking like they normally would, as if they were watching the game in the bonus room at home. It occurred to me at that moment that THAT is what love is. Not always a feeling, but always a commitment. My oldest brother once told me that you can't just be committed to the person; you have to be committed to the marriage, because you're not always going to feel in love with your spouse, and you're not always going to feel committed to them. You have to believe that the marriage is greater than the sum of its individuals.

My parents LOVE each other. I so much admire their strength and courage—for sticking with it through the toughest of times and for being the unwavering bedrock of what has to be one of the best families in the world. So here's to you, Mom and Dad, my heroes, and to many more. Thank you. For everything.

Happy Anniversary. And in the words of the great Harvey Lindenthal Cosper, Jr., "Let's all line up and get root canals in honor of the occasion." #dadquote

Becoming More Dependent

More than nine months after the stroke, we had finally settled into a routine of sorts. Harvey was living at home, walking with a cane, gingerly navigating the stairs to our bedroom at night, using our shower in the mornings, getting dressed with some help, eating normal food for the most part, and trying to exercise a little. For a while, we were able to get out to restaurants, appointments, and even to cheer at one of our grandson's basketball games at the YMCA without extra help. I kept a small, borrowed wheelchair in the back of my SUV in case we needed it for longer distances, and Harvey could use a walker, although it was difficult with his weak left arm and hand. But I could never even run out to the grocery store or take a walk unless someone was at the house with him.

I began to research options for reliable help. I chose a professional company that provided training, guaranteed presence during the specified hours, and insurance to cover any incidents or accidents involving their employees. Over time, we did employ several good independent caregivers, as well. Agency rates were somewhat higher, with a minimum of four hours per visit, but they guaranteed someone would be there even if our regularly assigned helper were unable to come. Harvey's caregiver was a man who shared his interest in sports, cars, and fishing. For many months, Randy came twice a week for four hours so that I could get out of the house for workouts, errands, appointments, and time with friends. Randy helped Harvey with his shower and dressing, as well as exercises for his left hand and practice with walking. They sometimes went out to breakfast together.

Meanwhile, the care team visits continued on Thursday nights. When Ann was home for the weekend, or when friends were available to help at the curb, Harvey was able to get to church while I sang in the choir. Once we even tried going to a movie; but, par for the course, the experience did not work out well. With his limited vision and difficulty walking, Harvey and I finally got seated and situated, and then an employee entered the theatre and announced to everyone that the movie would be showing in a different theatre. By the time we groped through the dim light down several steps with our popcorn, drinks, Harvey, and his walker and found our way through the dark to the other room, the movie was well underway. We stayed to the end, though, and, on the way out, I told the ticket-taker about our experience. As we inched our way back toward the parking lot, an employee ran after us waving two complimentary tickets. Unfortunately, we did not feel comfortable trying to return. Harvey and I both were having difficulty focusing on long shows, anyway. I suspected that would be our last movie outing together.

    I tried signing him up for all kinds of activities to pique his interest: a painting class, workouts with a trainer, swimming at the local aquatics center, and volunteering to serve homeless guests at Room in the Inn. But everything was such an effort for him, and only the trainer sessions worked out long-term. Harvey was not able to make much progress, but he tried. One day, as he inched along the track, hugging the railing at the church gym, the trainer stretched out her tape measure and announced that he had walked a few feet farther than the last session. He responded, "Catch me if you can."

    We had many doctor appointments and, when prescribed, more physical therapy sessions. Getting in and out of the car was difficult, as was my pushing the wheelchair up the ramp into the house, and more than once I had to enlist neighbors or work crews on the street to help us. We continued seeing our friendly paramedics and firemen who responded to the falls. Sometimes the injuries required hospitalization, especially when the medics saw the amount of blood that flowed each time from a patient on blood thinners. It was difficult keeping up with the the medications, the wrappings on his deteriorating skin, the persistent rashes and pain from the Sweet's Syndrome, and occasional infections.

To cut down on our trips to the cardiology clinic, a home health nurse trained me to test Harvey's blood for the clotting factor—a weekly necessity given the blood thinners he had to take to reduce the chance of another stroke. But I was truly inept. Harvey politely tried to hide his trepidation whenever I wielded the finger-pricking device; I usually made several attempts before getting just the right amount of blood on just the right part of the circle on the test strip while remembering to push just the right buttons at the right time. Wound care specialists taught me how to care for his skin tears. Fortunately, I was better at this task. We had to order expensive non-stick wound materials that arrived regularly in the mail; each precious square had to be carefully cut to cover each different wound, then wrapped in non-stick white strips. This task I performed well and proudly.

During this relatively quiet time at home, we made a number of professional appointments we had neglected during the preceding months. We upgraded his hearing aids. The ophthalmologists who had treated Harvey for glaucoma and retinal folds confirmed that he had lost total vision in one eye

—probably from a stroke in the optic nerve. With that and his left-side neglect, Harvey now qualified as legally blind. Even with this devastating news, we joked about having our ancient little dachshund Hank trained as a seeing-eye dog. Harvey was fitted for new glasses to improve vision in the other eye, and we enrolled at the Metrolina Association for the Blind, where the staff was helpful with strategies for reading, scanning, and locating objects—even though Harvey continued to ask them when he could drive again. On these occasions, the doctor and I would make eye contact with looks of regret. I repeated: "The doctor hasn't cleared you yet. Let's wait till you are moving around a little better."

The dermatologist wanted to start him on a new protocol for the Sweet's but, with everything else going on, we declined. The rheumatologist who had treated the Sweet's Syndrome for years continued to tweak medications to try to control the flares that never stopped coming. I just kept wondering how Harvey could cope with all this—it seemed everything was falling apart.

One day I was in the kitchen preparing a favorite recipe: sausage balls. As Harvey sat on the stool at the island, I thought that his old job of rolling the dough into balls would be a diversion as well as good practice for his weakened hand. He had liked cooking and always been meticulous in working with his hands. I was surprised, and heartbroken, to see that he rolled the balls into widely different sizes, some tiny, some large, most too loosely packed, as he placed them on the pan. This demonstrated a problem not just with dexterity and vision, but with perception in his injured brain.

Harvey was different in other ways, too, since the last time he had lived at home. He continued to lose weight. His left hand was nearly useless, and he had to use his right arm to lift his left arm. Reading continued to be difficult and exhausting—even when I drew heavy black lines down the left side of each page to remind him to scan all the way back before starting another line. This also affected his ability to write, even to sign his name legibly—which, arguably, he had not done even before the stroke. He wasn't interested in doing much. Most of all, he missed his work. He needed to feel needed.

Others in the law firm had taken over his clients and all of his cases. He continued to inquire about them, but, in an effort to spare him any worry, the younger partners, associates, paralegals, and secretaries carried on without much advice from him. After so many months, it was becoming obvious that his career had come to an end.

CHAPTER 11

THE GOODBYES BEGIN

Some people are predisposed to gratitude. Some are naturally better than others at it. But we all have to work on it... Giving thanks in the middle of things helps us get through them. It's a matter of grit and willpower, a defiant act: we will give thanks, anyway. We can choose the complaint of the weary or the joy of the thankful.

Dr. Robert W. Henderson,
"In All Circumstances?" sermon series:
"With Grateful Hearts," Covenant Presbyterian Church,
March 3, 2019

One day in early winter, about nine months after the stroke, a technology expert from the law firm came to our home to set up Harvey's computer and dictating equipment in an upstairs bedroom we had converted to an office. Harvey could not remember the passwords and procedures, so we placed informative sticky notes on the screens. The staffer pretended not to notice a huge dent in the wall of that room made by Harvey's head from an earlier fall.

A few mornings later, Harvey announced that he was going upstairs to do some work. I felt nervous and fearful as I imagined him at the desk. Even the simplest task of reaching to open a file folder would be difficult using just one hand. The house was quiet. I busied myself with laundry and other jobs that took me past the room in which he was working, without appearing to hover.

After several hours we ate a quiet lunch and, obviously exhausted, Harvey took a long nap. That evening, I heard him say to our daughter on the phone, "I tried to work some today." There was a silence in which I expect Ann was responding, "How did it go?" And then I heard him say, "I'm done."

February 16, 2014
From: Harvey (dictated to Kandy)
To: (three younger attorneys in his department)
Subject: Meeting
Gentlemen:

I need to speak with the three of you fairly soon about my current status with the firm and future plans. I would appreciate your placing a call to me for this purpose. Could the three of you propose a time this week when you would be available? Generally, early morning or after 4:00 p.m. is best for me.

Thanks. I look forward to speaking with you.
Harvey

The Goodbyes Begin

March 15, 2014
From: Kandy
Subject: Harvey's news

In a letter to the board of directors of the law firm, Harvey has submitted his notice of retirement from the practice of law effective March 31, 2014. He says that he has enjoyed every minute of his career. It has become clear to him that, even though he made significant progress during rehabilitation from his stroke nearly a year ago, he can no longer work as he has done for the past thirty-eight years.

This is not a Hallmark moment for "congratulations on entering a new phase of life." Harvey would have preferred to retire when he was ready, on his own, a few years from now. He would prefer to have the ability to enjoy retirement as he had imagined, doing things that are difficult now, like fishing, boating, tinkering with cars, reading, and traveling.

I am proud of his long, successful career and the respect he has earned in the legal, insurance, and medical professions and beyond. Harvey would not reveal it himself, but his colleagues affirm that he has established a legacy in litigation in this state for diligence, fairness, integrity, courtesy, and intelligence. In every medical institution in which he was incarcerated last year, doctors and staff flocked in to speak to him and thank him for all he had done for them.

We are sad today. We face challenges. Harvey will

> *continue to work at regaining strength and developing new interests.*
>
> *We are grateful for our children, our friends, and our church family. We are grateful for his caregiver, Randy, who helps in whatever ways he is needed, and for our care team, who are fun for Harvey and who give me the opportunity to spend time with friends and sing. We are grateful for friends who have continued to let us know they care, who go out to eat with us and come for visits. We are grateful for our comfortable home in Charlotte and for our place in Wilmington, which gives us a change of scenery and another wonderful group of friends.*
>
> *We enjoy invitations to get together with people, together or separately. We enjoy visits, and we love hearing from you!*
>
> *Most of all, we are grateful for our faith in the goodness of God, who carries us always, on the bad days and the good.*

Thankfully, this would be my last emailed update for a year—a time in which we continued to live a life of highs and lows, celebrations and pain. As always, we lived in that world of contradictory realities in which I was never unwary, after a good day, that a bad day was likely to follow. I did not comprehend it then, but we were living a long series of goodbyes.

As we neared the first anniversary of the stroke, we were offered a special gift by my sister and her husband: they invited Harvey to stay with them for a weekend while I had some relaxing time to myself. I discovered an historic bed and breakfast inn near their lovely horse farm in rural Durham County and counted the days until time to go. We were understandably anxious about the difficulties they might encounter with Harvey, but I was exhausted in every way, and it would be good for us to have a couple of days apart.

Unfortunately, the two-hour car trip to their home was a disaster. First, we had a bathroom emergency. We were rescued by a large, gentle male attendant at a rest area off I-85. He saw that we were in trouble, and he stayed with us, helping in every way. Then, not long after we got back on the highway, Harvey threw up in the car.

By the time Harvey was settled at Jan and Bob's and I made my way to the B&B, it was long past check-in and the dinner served to guests. But after taking my small bag to a cozy bedroom, the owner showed me to a table in the empty dining room with a place that was set just for me. Fresh flowers, fine china, a linen napkin, a delicious home-cooked meal, a cold glass of wine, and a scrumptious dessert awaited me. When I finally climbed the creaking wooden stairs back to my room, a gas fire flickered in the fireplace. In my four-poster bed, I fell asleep with a novel barely touched at my side and a stain of tears on my pillowcase.

Most of the following day was spent in locating and patronizing a business that could clean the vomit and disinfect the seats and rugs in my Toyota. I did get in a short hike in the afternoon. It was wonderful to be alone, to rest and think and pray in a quiet place. I met and discovered connections with interesting people at breakfast and dinner and slept well both nights.

The Defense Rests

When I returned to pick up Harvey the following morning, he had just fallen on his face. Only his glasses were broken—no bones. We reassured Bob and Jan that this was par for the course and they were not to feel responsible for it in the least. They expressed gratitude that their red oriental rug would not show blood stains. And then we drove home, appreciating them, appreciating each other, and appreciating the fact that we made the entire two-hour trip back with no catastrophes.

The following week, I sent an email to the state highway department commending the employee who had assisted us with such patience and care at the rest area. Many months later, when I happened to stop there again—alone—I saw the man and thanked him again. He insisted he was just doing his job, but I knew better.

April 13, 2014
Ann's Facebook Post

In one hour will be the first anniversary of when Mom came upstairs during the neighborhood party to check on my sleeping dad only to find him halfway out of the bed and partially paralyzed from a stroke. In some ways it feels like it's been years and, in other ways, it still feels like a dream.

I am so proud of my parents' strength and determination day-in and day-out. The past few months have been tough ones. Dad has had to retire due to the seemingly never-ending physical and mental challenges. But he is now working on using his cane less, and things seem to be looking up. He was in great spirits when I was waxing philosophical about the significance of this day, telling me, "I'm afraid to go take a nap!" And then he told me a dirty joke. Love that guy.

#dadquote

- Me: "How are you, Dad?"

Dad: "I'm good. Well, I say I'm good, but your mom is wielding surgical scissors and I'm scared to death."

- My eight-year-old nephew, on Dad's health: "Granddaddy used to be an athlete but he had a stroke and now he's a commentator on SportsCenter."

A GRATEFUL NATION

Early in the summer of 2014, another event confirmed for us that we were living a life of sharp contrasts, of blessing and misfortune, love and loss. I saw my husband both as the frail man he had become and the strong man he always would be. It reinforced that **it is important for people who develop disabilities to be regarded and recognized as the same people they always were.**

As we had done for many years, we drove to a resort on Hilton Head Island in South Carolina for the annual meeting of the North Carolina Association of Defense Attorneys, a group in which Harvey had been a long-time leader. Assisted by my sister and my daughter—both lawyers—we attended the gathering of women and men who had been colleagues and friends for decades. Only this time we took a cane and a wheelchair. I knew that Harvey's long-time friends would be shocked by his appearance and his condition. To my chagrin, in a group known for khakis and golf shirts, he insisted on wearing a flowered Hawaiian shirt and a broad-brimmed straw hat to the opening reception while sporting a grizzly beard. Beaming, Ann told him that he looked great and he responded, "I know."

During the first morning's convocation of more than three hundred attorneys and judges, Harvey was introduced by a friend and former law partner who described his reputation and career success and gentlemanly ways, mentioning his humility, kindness and compassion, intellect and understanding of the law, his sense of humor, mentoring of younger lawyers, and his dedication to his clients and to his profession. The speaker talked about Harvey's induction a few years earlier into the American College of Trial Lawyers, which accepts fewer than one percent of trial lawyers nationwide; then he listed some other accolades that I never even knew about. After that, Harvey was called up to the stage to receive the organization's award for "exemplifying the highest standards of professionalism, integrity and ethics while conducting himself in a courteous and civil manner."

Everyone in the room stood, applauding. As colleagues balanced his frail arms on either side, Harvey moved ever so slowly up the steps and across the stage. Finally, he stood at the lectern and looked out over the crowd. I felt queasy. He had no prepared written remarks—he could not physically have written or read them, anyway. His brain worked differently now. He looked so tall and gaunt, grizzled, his face crooked from the stroke, his skin mottled, his hair thin and white. I prayed that he would be able to speak, that he would not embarrass himself, and that his colleagues would still see the dignified and respected attorney he had always been instead of a pitiful, broken, handicapped old man.

The room grew quiet. Harvey joked about having taken so long to make his way to the podium. As we all held our breath, he stood silently as though he had all the time in the world. Finally, in slow, deep and careful tones, he began to talk. Haltingly but determinedly, he asked the audience to look around them and see some of the best lawyers in the country. He said that he was "just a plodder" who had loved every single minute of his work. He referred to "that little silver-haired lady over there" who had cared for the home and family to make it possible for him to do what he did, looked over at me and added, "Thank you, Honey." Between pauses, he told a couple of funny stories about trials. He ended with, "As the saying goes, on behalf of a grateful nation, thank you."

While his colleagues stood and clapped again, even longer this time, I saw that this beloved man, who never wanted any recognition or awards of any kind, was truly and justly proud. He was still the revered gentleman who had graced courtrooms across the region. And that day we could add one more adjective: he was brave.

When he finally made his way back to his seat, someone handed me the pointed glass sculpture with inscription. Quoting a favorite movie, *A Christmas Story,* Harvey looked it over and declared with a crooked smile, "It's a major award!"

Once we arrived home, our celebratory mood did not last long. One morning soon afterward, Harvey fell while leaving a restaurant, which he renamed the IDrop, with his caregiver. For weeks after that, he was in pain from several broken ribs, for which there was no cure except time. It was then that we realized the damage done to his bones by the high doses of steroids he had taken over the years. He had begun to experience pain in his back from a disc fracture that made it harder for him to sit up. We were using a wheelchair more often, and I was poorly equipped to help him transfer, even with help from the caregiver. He considered having an outpatient procedure to relieve pain by filling the disc fracture with cement-like material.

Meanwhile, his closest law partner and friend hosted a retirement party for Harvey. He enjoyed the many jokes and stories shared by lawyers and co-workers from across the state and told a few himself. The group presented him with a framed Bible verse, Micah 6:8, signed around the edges by those in attendance, that they felt described the way Harvey lived his life: *"What does the Lord require of you but to do justice, love mercy, and walk humbly with your God."*

By October, Harvey had been living at home for nearly a year. Many people had helped us in many ways. In gratitude, one evening we entertained a small group of special people who had helped us most, all in different but important ways. We sat outside on the same porch as the neighborhood party eighteen months earlier on the day of the stroke. We served an Italian supper and a cake adorned with "We love our friends!" in bright red script. As they left, we gave each guest a loaf of homemade pumpkin bread. Such paltry offerings for such extravagant expressions of love. This followed the theme Harvey had set from the first day of illness: let those who help you know how grateful you are.

It was the first party we had given since that terrible night—and the last we would ever give together.

Ten days later, he was in the orthopedic hospital for outpatient surgery on his back.

October 21, 2014
Ann's Facebook Post

Dad update: My dad has been dealing with a spinal compression fracture, which has been very painful and has made things significantly more difficult for him and for my little spitfire mom who tirelessly takes care of him around the clock. He had surgery this morning to relieve some of the pressure on his spinal cord, and everything went well. He feels great right now, but of course he's still a little doped up, so it's too early to tell whether this will provide substantial long-term relief. When I spoke with him just now, he quoted one of his favorite movies, "Analyze This": "Pain? Gone. Where is it? Don't know." #dadquote

Thank you for all the prayers and support!

December 21, 2014
Ann's Facebook Post
#dadquote

- *On our appetizer: "Somewhere there are a bunch of frogs walking around on crutches."*
- *On talking to himself: "It's the only time anyone*

around here will listen."
- *On a football player trying to run: "Looks like he is pulling a piano."*
- *On a UNC basketball player: "They're pushing him around like a broom out there." (Another fantastic broom metaphor: "Looks like Coach Roy pulled him out of his broom closet.")*

"End stage": a tough call

When I look back now at the end of 2014, I can see how debilitated and miserable Harvey had become. But gradual decline is difficult to see when you are with a person every day. Love and hope can serve as blinders. It took an unexpected intervention to force me to face the truth.

In early December, Graham had taken his dad to pick out a Christmas tree for us while I went for a haircut. As I was sitting in the salon chair with wet hair, my cell phone announced a call from the hospital. Excusing myself, I moved to a sunny bench in the lobby to answer.

Harvey's experienced physical therapist, who had worked with him many times over the preceding eighteen months, opened the conversation by saying that she cared very much for us; that she prayed for her patients every day and felt a special bond with us. That she hoped she was not overstepping her boundaries with this call. She felt led, however, to tell me what she was seeing in my husband.

"I worked with Mr. Cosper back in January," she said, "and then again in November—and the decline during that time is shocking. He is debilitated. He has lost muscle mass. He is frail and fragile. He has the body of an eighty-year-old man. I think it's important for you to understand that he is in the end stage...."

End stage. We let the words rest between us. I didn't ask, "End of what?"

"I'm not saying he is going to die tomorrow, or next month," she said. "You have done a wonderful job of encouraging and pushing him to get better, and this doesn't mean that you need to stop. But you might think about how you want to handle things from here. His deterioration is a process that is going to continue." (Pause.) "I felt you needed to know."

I had a hard time breathing. I felt leaden and cold. I thanked her for calling, said I knew it had been hard for her and I appreciated her honesty. We disconnected. I swam above myself and saw that I was sitting in a bright room with plants, and people were chatting nearby, and why was I there?

Like a robot, I paid the hairdresser and escaped into the crisp air with my hair still wet.

Back at home, Graham was helping his dad into bed for a rest. We joked that he had taken better care of his dad than the last time he'd come over; that time, I had returned to find the two of them in a jolly mood on the back porch drinking brown liquid from highball glasses and eating potato chips for lunch. Now, with Harvey asleep, we settled into chairs in the den, redolent with pine resin from a tree draped with colored lights in the corner, and I told our son about the phone call. He looked at me with sadness and perhaps a little bit of guilt: he had already known. In fact, he had always known, from the moment of the stroke twenty months earlier. And the truth is that, for some months, I had known, too.

It was then that Graham revealed to me what the neurosurgeon said on the night of the stroke: his father would likely end up in a nursing home. And as a physician, Graham had a clear view of the truth.

"It must have been a very lonely feeling to be Graham," Ann told me later, "because he knew from the beginning. He didn't want to discourage anyone, take anyone's hope away. There is no other man he will ever love more than his dad.

"You were more optimistic than perhaps was reasonable," she continued. "But, Mom, you push people. And we decided you needed to be that way. If you didn't truly believe Dad could get better, you wouldn't have pushed him as you did. And he might not have improved as much or lived as long."

The following week, on December 19, the customary long-stemmed red roses were delivered to our house with a wedding anniversary card that read, "*For Kandy – My loving wife, my best friend, mother of three great children, and my best care provider. With all my love and profound appreciation, Harvey.*"

Over the next twelve months, we were to face seven more hospitalizations, three moves to other facilities that nobody wanted to make, and another anniversary that changed our family forever. On that day, he would call out to me, but I wouldn't hear him.

The Goodbyes Begin

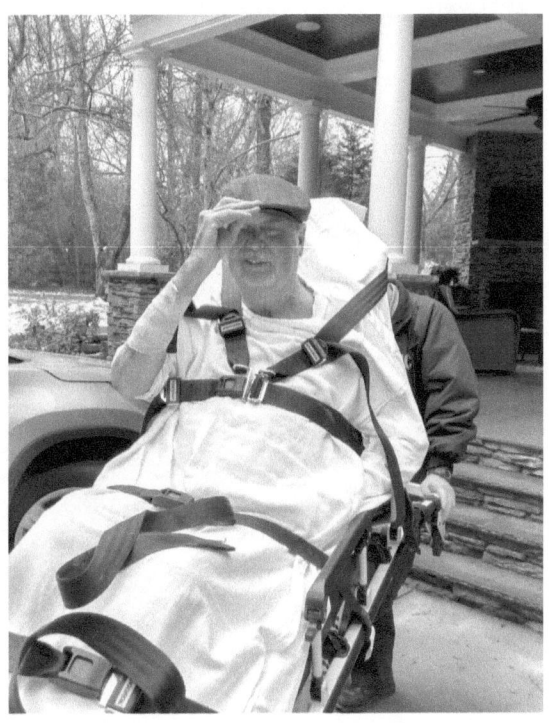

PART 3

WHEN ILLNESS DIVIDES THE HOME

God's usual way of working in the world to alleviate suffering, injustice, and pain is not to intervene miraculously, suspending the laws of nature, violating the principles of human freedom, or sending angels to make things right. No, God works through people. God sees, hears, and knows the suffering of others. God expects his people to do the same. And God's response is to call us to step up as instruments of his aid.

Adam Hamilton,
Moses: In the Footsteps of the Reluctant Prophet

Chapter 12

Losing Our Options

Give me the strength to lightly bear my joys and sorrows.
                                               Rabindranath Tagore

Looking back, my image of Harvey on his last Christmas with us is one of wistfulness and resignation. He seems to be receding to the edges of the picture. On Christmas Eve, David ably assumed his dad's place in the kitchen, making the roast beef and gravy, as Graham gathered up the crumpled wrapping paper and bows. The clear picture in my mind is this: in the hubbub of children and grandchildren, visitors, cookies, decorations, enticing aromas, and presents under the tree, Harvey sits quietly in his favorite armchair. He listens to classical music on the Davidson College radio station. He leans his head back and closes his eyes. His large frame is skinny and frail. He has grown a short, scraggly white beard because shaving is too difficult. His hands and arms are blue, red, and black where not covered in bandages, while his cheeks and forehead are mottled with the ever-present rash. He smiles, but he doesn't say much. *What is he thinking? Is he feeling left out? Is he making a long, slow transition from the everyday world in which he used to play such a vibrant part?*

He continued to be grateful and undemanding. He continued to make funny comments. He knew what was going on around him and interacted in his quiet way. As always, he spoke to God with a beautiful blessing at the table. The grandchildren sat on his lap. But he seemed exhausted and sad. He went to bed early.

Meanwhile, I am asking myself, *How long can I continue to care for him at home? Should I spend the money to hire more caregiving time? If so, where will the person sleep? Will my husband have to move into some kind of nursing home? No. No! Should we both move to a retirement place? Could we afford it? But where? He's only sixty-six! To one of those places in which the urine-scented halls are lined with desiccated old people slumped in wheelchairs, calling for help? Sharing a room with a stranger, eating tasteless food, being forced into diapers? How can I do that to him? But how am I going to keep looking after him at home when it is starting to take more than one person to help him through the day?*

He was brave and accepting. He did not want pity. But we were losing control. We were running out of options. And I was filled with fear.

March 1, 2015
To: choir director
From: Kandy
Subject: missing choir again

  I won't be at choir because Harvey is back in the hospital with small back fractures and left side weakness. He had two falls in two hours on Friday. Will have to go through rehab again but we are determined to bring him home to live. Sorry this message is late.

March 1, 2015
Ann's Facebook Post

Dad Facetimed me from the hospital to tell me he has two more compression fractures in his back. Then he said that was the late "breaking" (get it?) news and he had to go because "Downton Abbey" was on. Love that guy.

#dadquote

- "If at first you don't succeed, don't try skydiving."

March 5, 2015
From: Kandy
Subject: Harvey is at it again

During the year since I last sent out an update, Harvey has stayed out of the hospital and we have managed okay at home with minimal help from a wonderful caregiver. We have attended church, enjoyed meals with friends, and even traveled to the beach a few times. However, he has gradually lost a good bit of his strength and endurance. In October, he had outpatient surgery to relieve pain from a compression fracture in his back. Then recently, during February, he lost the use of his left hand altogether and began dragging his left foot. He had two more painful back fractures and many skin tears.

Last Friday, we called 911 twice in two hours to get

him up from falls and finally sent him by ambulance to the hospital. While there, he began having issues with heart rhythm. Once again, there is consternation over what to do about blood thinners in a person who's had a stroke but who also could hit his head in a fall.

Today, he was transported to a new hospital rehabilitation center. For the next couple of weeks, they will evaluate Harvey's issues and try to help him regain some strength. They will also help us learn how we can best keep him safe at home. I expect we will be hiring some more help.

Harvey continues to be just as smart, funny, and kind as he ever was. But he is so tired and uncomfortable. Please pray with us that this—the fourth complete stint in rehab in less than two years—will give him, and us, a better quality of life and the ability to remain in our home together. We send our love to each of you and to your families.

A perfect emailed response from a friend:

Dear Kandy, You and Harvey have gone through so much and remain cheerful and optimistic. I'm just so sorry that this is happening again and pray that his condition will improve. You know we are here for you. Lots of love.

P.S. Later today I will drop in the mail a card directly to Harvey at rehab. Please let us know when visits are encouraged. Thanks.

March 12, 2015
Ann's Facebook Post
#dadquote
- When Kandy Cosper commented on the giant bowl of grits he ate this morning, my dad said, "I got grit-faced."

March 3, 2015
From: Kandy
Subject: re: Harvey is at it again

The Tar Heels let us down last night, but I am attaching a photo we posted on Facebook to demonstrate that we held up our end over here. Photo caption: "If I get in trouble, are you going to kick me out?" (Photo of Harvey in a hospital bed, in a chip frenzy, with a bottle and a cup filled with yellow-gold liquid)

We will find out on Tuesday what the goals are for Harvey's improvement during his stay, along with his expected release date in a couple of weeks. This is a lovely new facility, quiet with great employees, good food, large rooms, and a glassed-in atrium for sunny days. Harvey seems to be doing better—which could be from raising his low B12 level with injections. In PT yesterday, he actually walked 165 feet with his cane!

Please don't feel you have to do anything for us—we are doing okay. But if you do plan on sending a card, it will get to him faster with the address of the rehab facility. While he is so well cared for, I am taking a few days at the *coast from Wednesday to Sunday. Ann will be here for the weekend. If anyone is interested in dropping in on Harvey at the ALC Wednesday or Thursday around dinnertime, please let me know ahead of time. For the weekend, Ann can be reached… Thanks for all your messages—we read every one aloud and enjoy them!*

Harvey says "thanks for your continued thoughts and prayers." P.S. The liquid in the cup came from the bottle.

"What Am I Doing?"

Harvey's fourth inpatient rehab stint in two years, with efficient doctors and therapists who had not worked with him before, seemed a good place to reassess whether he had the ability to improve his mobility and increase his independence. He actually seemed to improve overall and was walking pretty well with a cane. But when he returned home about two weeks later, he could not get in and out of bed without more help than I could give. When he needed to get up in the middle of the night, I got up with him, but sometimes he toppled to the floor. Medics came several times to help. Almost overnight, managing stairs became even more difficult. It became impossible to take him to outside appointments.

When Harvey transferred to the new downstairs bedroom, with its smaller bed and raised head, I couldn't leave him alone to sleep. He still needed help turning over, getting to the bathroom, even pulling himself up by the bedrail. We began using the wheelchair inside the house more often. He seemed to grow weaker by the day. No one could figure out what was happening, or why. Since I wasn't getting much rest, several times I hired a nighttime caregiver who slept on the floor of his room so that I could go upstairs for a few hours of sleep.

Ann, David, and Graham had remained, as always, respectful of our decisions throughout all the challenging months. They never told us what to do. They asked good questions and supported us always. But I could tell from their expressions of concern that they felt their dad's time of living at home was coming to an end. He had been hospitalized on February 27, March 4, March 23, and April 3, for one to fifteen days each time.

Around-the-clock home care was not a good option for us, since Harvey needed at least two helpers in order to transfer. Perhaps I could be trained to manage more of his needs, but his left side was dead weight. I tended to become impatient and panic when we got stuck. More than once I exploded in frustration during difficult situations and falls—"This is terrible! I can't do it!"—always followed by guilt and remorse as he remained quiet and helpless. We just couldn't go on like this.

With a heart so heavy I had to take deep breaths, I began to research inpatient care facilities. A new assisted living center (ALC) was under construction just a block from our house, but it was not due to open for a few months. During a visit to the sales office, I discovered that the company had completed a new facility south of town, about twenty-five minutes away, where

Harvey could live until the new building opened nearby. Then I could just walk over to spend time with him. It sounded so good that, once again, my optimism overtook my judgment. At the time, I didn't know the difference between assisted living and skilled nursing; it didn't occur to me to ask whether they provided skilled nursing care when residents needed it. As we learned the hard way, they did not.

I tried to talk to Harvey about his moving to the ALC. Surely he didn't want to leave our home of thirty years? Adjust to a new place with a bunch of strangers taking care of him, surrounded by residents twenty years older than he? But he did not object. When I told him that I just couldn't care for him at home any more, that it was no longer safe, he was calm and accepting, as though he understood. He said he was ready to go.

I will never know how much of his acquiescence stemmed from his natural kindness and love for me; how much was truly his judgment that this was for the best, or how much was his way of just giving up. But I filled out the forms and submitted a deposit for a one-bedroom apartment. We drove out for a personal meeting, evaluation, and tour of the facility. Harvey was accepted for assisted living. Once again, my friend who is an interior designer helped me assess the space and select furnishings using pieces from the new room at home. I purchased single bedding and a comfortable lift chair, then packed some of his clothes. As I folded the soft white undershirts, socks, sweat pants, toiletries, and family photos into suitcases, I kept thinking, *"What in the world am I doing?"*

May 7, 2015
Kandy's Facebook Post

So, while the caregiver was with Harvey this morning, I was rushing home to unpack a carload of purchases from Walmart, change clothes, and get to a Bible study group luncheon with my usual homemade pound cake. But I was delayed by tree trimmers blocking Sardis Road. Finally unloading at home, I realized that a bed pillow and the new seventy-dollar cover for Harvey's car must still be in the bottom of my cart in the Walmart parking lot. I drove back to the store but saw no carts in the lot with yellow car cover boxes in the bottom. Running in to customer service, I found that someone had turned in the pillow but not the box. "Can you believe someone would steal from a poor guy who had a stroke and can't drive his car?" I asked. A lot of people in line were interested in this. When I went to get another one and brought it back to customer service, the manager said, "You don't need to get back in line, Ma'am. Just take it with you." I thanked her very much and left. On the way to my car, I passed the yellow box lying on the path to the parking lot. I went back in to the service desk and sheepishly returned the box. Not to be foiled again by the flagman on Sardis Road, I detoured to Monroe and Rama. And that's where I stopped for the train.

The Defense Rests

Choosing a Care Facility

During that spring and summer, I learned a lot about retirement facilities and nursing homes.

- **Senior independent living communities are sprouting as healthy older adults look to down-size from their houses and live without responsibility for home maintenance.** These apartment-style and cottage-style complexes offer a variety of amenities and activities to enhance life in the later years. While they are still relatively healthy and mobile, seniors can choose their level of activity and involvement, make new friends, and continue to enjoy the wider communities and towns in which they live.
- **Assisted living facilities are for residents who can perform the basic activities of daily living with minimal (one-person assist) help.** This includes bathing, grooming, dressing, eating, toileting, ambulating, and transferring themselves, as from bed to chair or wheelchair. Their staffs include certified nursing assistants (CNAs) who are trained to assist residents but are not allowed to physically lift them, for obvious reasons of safety for both the patients and the caregivers. Some wheelchair-bound patients can get along fine in assisted living, because they have the ability to transfer themselves with minimal help. Each extra service required, including the administration of medications, can add to the monthly fees. Many assisted living residences offer special memory care services or units. They can also offer inpatient rehabilitation that is

either limited to patients already residing in the facility or open to temporary patients from the outside.
- **Skilled nursing units typically provide services for rehabilitation patients who need professional care for a specific medical need, such as post-surgery recovery.** They do not need the high-level, extensive medical care provided by hospitals, but they require more nursing assistance than assisted living facilities offer. Patients are admitted following medical events from which they expect to improve.
- **Nursing homes provide round-the-clock custodial care for patients with physical or mental disabilities who cannot live on their own, necessitating permanent nursing care and assistance with activities of daily living.** Memory care is generally included.
- **A fourth category of residential options for seniors is the continuing care retirement community (CCRC).** These senior communities offer residents a continuum of care, from independent living to assisted living to rehabilitation to skilled nursing/healthcare, and most have memory care units as well. They offer lodging—rooms, apartments, and cottages—as well as meals, laundry and cleaning services, hairdressers, exercise options, entertainment, outings, and social activities. They have nurses, CNAs, and doctors on staff. Once you pay the entry fee, you can move from one area to another as required by your health status and, as long as you pay the monthly charges based on how much care you receive, you will never have to leave. Depending

on space availability—years-long waiting lists are not uncommon—most CCRCs reserve their skilled nursing spaces for their own residents who might need them. Continuing care facilities are options only for people who have substantial assets or, for those needing skilled nursing, long-term care insurance.

May 8, 2015
Ann's Facebook Post

Facebook friends: After being taken care of for over two years since his stroke by my amazing, unsinkable mother, next Thursday, the big guy is moving to, as he calls it, the "old folks' home." No one expects to be sixty-six years old when this happens, but it has, and it is the only way to keep Dad safe at this point. As Dad says, "It's not the best possible situation, but it's the best situation possible." Of course, he already has hilarious stories about meeting his "fellow inmates," as he calls them, and I know there are going to be so many more legendary #dadquotes to come. And Kandy Cosper is already scoping out her competition at Dad's new home because, let's be honest —the man is pretty darn charming. Please pray for us as we transition into this new phase in the life of our family. #dadquote

- I hear this joke every year: "Hey Ann, when is Mother's Day?"

"I don't know, Dad. When?"

"Nine months after Father's Day."

May 9, 2015
From: Harvey (as dictated to Kandy)

Dear Friends:

Time to go to the old folks' home. Next Thursday, May 14, I will be moving to a retirement center (a euphemism for old folks' home). The plan is to transfer to their closer location when it opens this fall. Our house of thirty years here will always be home, and I will be here a lot. We also plan to continue to spend time at the coast when we can. But I hope you will come visit me at my home away from home. I can always be reached on my cell phone. I can also be reached through Kandy. Come on out for a game of shuffleboard.

Best to everyone,
Harvey

Chapter 13

The End of Living Together

Some days there won't be a song in your heart. Sing anyway.
                                                    Emory Austin

Moving Day

On May 14, two years and one month after the stroke, I filled my SUV with clothes, toiletries, plants, framed pictures, linens, and a few kitchen items before driving out to set up Harvey's apartment. Movers delivered the few larger furnishings. Friends came out to help me set it all up. It looked nice. Harvey arrived with Randy that afternoon.

I wondered how my husband was feeling that day as he was driven from the home in which he had lived with his family for thirty years—as he was rolled, helpless, into an apartment in a building full of strangers. But we just didn't talk about it. We were keeping him safer. We were keeping me safer, and saner. We were doing what had to be done.

The truth is that I was moving, too—just not sleeping there

overnight—and had, in a sense, been living away from home much of the time since the stroke. I had left him many nights in other places while I went home to sleep, only to return early the next morning to spend another day. But this time...this time was different, because we knew it was permanent.

What were we thinking? I asked myself over and over. All the forty-four years together, the thousands of days and nights together, all the love and the life and the memories, and he would never live at home again. *Why were we doing this?* Was there a "right thing" to do? How would he feel out there by himself in that narrow bed, night after night, with a button hanging from his neck to call a stranger when he needed something, while his wife and the place he had lived with his family for so many years was miles away in the darkness?

Returning home exhausted that night to our quiet house, I walked through the back door onto Harvey's porch, where the leaves of the star magnolia and cherry tree had formed a bower to the back yard. I ran my hand across the back of his favorite striped chair. I paced through the house, my wails the only sound. I touched his shirts and ties in the closet, a pair of reading glasses beside the bed, a brush with wisps of hair that smelled like him. His bathroom cup. His favorite cereal, his books and CDs, the pictures of the family all together over the years. His pillow on his side of our bed. The last towel that had dried his body after a shower.

I thought that I could not physically live with the pain that I felt. I thought that this was the saddest moment of my life.

The End of Living Together

When the Right Choice Is Not Right

The new ALC was lovely, but residents had been allowed to move in before it was finished, and there were kinks in the system. In Harvey's apartment, the kitchen sink was lying on the floor awaiting installation. Most importantly, the call system for aides and nurses was not working properly. Despite guarantees of a five-minute response time, Harvey sometimes waited more than hour for help getting to the bathroom or the bed, and I spent a lot of time roaming the halls seeking assistance. I had to be there to make sure he was transported to meals on time, therapists came as they were scheduled, nurses changed his dressings without using tape, his CPAP machine was hooked up at night, his medications and eye drops were current, and he was wheeled downstairs for activities that included Bible study and group crossword puzzles—although a lady in that group eventually asked Harvey to stop coming because he knew all the answers.

On the positive side, most of the staff was friendly, many of the other residents were interesting and engaged, the food and meal service were very good, and friends began to come out and visit Harvey in his comfortable new living room. These visits were the highlights of Harvey's days. The sweet lady next door couldn't carry on a conversation, but she banged away at some familiar old hymns on her piano at all hours, and we smiled about it. The young physical therapist was helpful and encouraging. We enjoyed visits with the aides when they had time to chat. In typical fashion, with his kind ways and gratitude for all they did for him, Harvey endeared himself to the staff, though I suspected some saw my vigilance on his behalf as interference. Again, we were grateful that proceeds from Harvey's disability policy would help us cover the expense for a while; when it ran out, we would need to begin liquidating our retirement investments.

Daily life began to smooth out. Spending most of every day with him, I maintained a whiteboard of therapy appointments and scheduled visits from friends, written in big colorful letters and propped where Harvey could see it. Several times I took him out to a restaurant close by for lunch, even though managing him with the wheelchair was difficult. The grandchildren painted pictures for the walls and we collected several plants he liked. Ann and I invited a few friends for a sixty-seventh birthday party for him, serving a bakery cake covered with fresh strawberries. We made new friends at meals in the dining room, and several interesting gentlemen ate with him whenever I wasn't there. At meals, though, Harvey never had much to say, and he (along with most of the other residents) had trouble hearing conversation from across the table. A couple of the female residents flirted with him and invited him to eat at their table. Once, as I passed through the hall, I smiled to overhear one of them exclaiming to another, "I saw Harvey today!"

Though he was still an interesting conversationalist and enjoyed his visitors, Harvey was increasingly more quiet and withdrawn, and he spent most of his time in the recliner in his room. As he grew weaker and thinner, he seemed to have more difficulty holding himself in a sitting position. He still enjoyed food, but eating was difficult—not just sitting up at the table, but also swallowing, as always, and handling implements. As the weeks passed, he began to request most of his meals in his room.

If he had a doctor appointment farther away than a few miles, we had to hire a special transport van, at considerable cost. The first time we did this, since our house was closer to the doctor's office, I made the mistake of choosing to meet Harvey at the appointment site, and the ALC staff made sure he boarded the van on time. But when the vehicle arrived at the clinic, I discovered Harvey in the back of the van, strapped in the wheelchair, slumped forward with his arms and head dangling to the floor. The driver informed me that he was not allowed to touch the patients he transported.

When he had been evaluated for admission to the facility, Harvey had apparently passed the requirements for ability to transfer with assistance from one person—between wheelchair and bed, lift chair, or shower chair. However, in the weeks following his admission, it became apparent that the CNAs were having difficulty with him. They were trying their best, they told us, but they were straining their backs. They began to call on one another for extra help, though two CNAs were rarely available at the same time given the standard nurse-to-patient ratio.

One day, one of the nurses informed me that, when a patient needs more than a one-person assist, guidelines for most facilities required the use of a lift. Harvey had been moved around in these Hoyer lifts a few times during past hospitalizations, and I had seen them outside the rooms of other patients at the ALC. I had observed that it often takes two nurses or therapists to maneuver patients into the lift, especially larger patients whose bodies are dead weight because they cannot help. Harvey had been experiencing significant back pain that further limited his mobility. The first time he was placed in the lift, he moaned as the nurses tried to wrap the thick canvas straps around him and hoist him into the air, swinging him high as head fell forward, while his bony legs and feet dangled below. His eyes were closed and he appeared defeated. I felt his discomfort and humiliation. I escaped into the hall and cried—not just that day, but every other time I saw it in the weeks that followed.

As the days stretched past the second full month there, the call button issues were resolved and Harvey settled into a routine. The staff obviously liked him and was taking good care of him. I decided to drive the four hours to the coast to check on our house for the first time in months. Graham would visit his dad when his schedule allowed, and I invited friends to drop in regularly in the two days before Ann arrived for the weekend. I wrote the schedule of activities and visitors on the whiteboard.

I had been away for forty-eight hours when the emergency call came: Harvey was being rushed to the hospital by ambulance. They feared he had become septic—an infection had reached his bloodstream. While I helped the dogs into the back of the car and headed back to Charlotte, a clammy and feverish Harvey was being carted off the premises in a stretcher.

One more place for him to leave and never see again.

July 19, 2015
Ann's Facebook Post

Update on the big guy: official diagnosis is that he had gotten septic as a result of a urinary tract infection.

The End of Living Together

So, so grateful for the big-time antibiotics that are working to keep my Dad "fogging the glass," as he would say. "It's not easy being Harvey Cosper, but someone's gotta do it." Fortunately, he's on the up and up and will hopefully be back at his apartment next week. Thank you everyone for your support! We appreciate it.

   #dadquote
   - Dad: "I'm not good at handling this phone anymore."
   Me: "To be fair, Dad, you were never good with technology. You can't blame everything on the stroke."
   Dad: "Yeah, I'm starting to think I've just always been slow."

No Place to Live

About eight weeks after he had moved to assisted living, and one week after he was sent to the hospital, Harvey's infection was successfully treated and doctors cleared him to be released. On a Thursday afternoon, I packed up his belongings and ordered a van to transport him back to his apartment at the ALC. To my shock, a hospital social worker hurried into the room to tell us that Harvey was not approved for re-admittance to the facility where he lived. I had not known that, after a hospitalization, the resident must be reassessed for admission as though he or she were a new applicant. The head of nursing at the ALC had stopped by earlier in the day, while I was out, and deemed Harvey unqualified to return. She left word that she was going to a conference out of town and would try to make another assessment in a week or so, although she was not confident that he would qualify even then.

Wait...what? The hospital is dismissing Harvey, but he can't go back to the place he lives? Then where is he supposed to go? And... right now, today?

The best way to describe my reaction that afternoon is that I absolutely lost it. In desperation, I tried to speak with the staff at both the hospital and the ALC. I begged the nurse manager to reconsider, or at least visit sooner for a second assessment. But they had no intention of taking Harvey back. They were not going to yield to the irrational request of the insistent wife: Mr. Cosper no longer met the qualifications for residency there. If we wanted to hold out hope that he could somehow improve enough to requalify in the weeks ahead, we could pay the $242 per day out-of-pocket to hold his room. Otherwise, we had a matter of days to vacate the apartment.

The problem with facilities offering only assisted living is that many, if not most, residents will at some time require higher levels of care—if not for permanent conditions, then for temporary ones: convalescence or rehabilitation following hospitalization for illness, surgery such as knee and hip replacement, or heart ailments, for example. If their residential facility does not offer skilled nursing, then they have to move again, either temporarily or permanently. Medicare will generally cover a certain number of doctor-prescribed days in rehab following hospitalization, while private insurance coverage may or may not be available. Meanwhile, patients must continue to pay for their rooms in the hope that they will improve enough to return.

My only choice was to select a skilled nursing facility, or nursing home, for subacute rehab and pray that Harvey's condition would improve enough for him to be re-admitted to the ALC. While I continued to pay for his ALC apartment, the nursing home fees would be covered by Medicare for a few weeks, as long as improvement could be documented. Unfortunately, no one was hopeful about that.

I did not blame the assisted living facility for their rules or for their decision; I knew that managing Harvey's needs was a hard job for those kind men and women who had tried to care for him. The two regrets I had were, first, their not making it clear to incoming residents that anyone needing skilled nursing would have to leave and, second, their not sitting down with us face to face to discuss, with patience and compassion, what they had decided and how we might proceed from there.

What I came to realize was that, for my part, I needed be in better control of myself. I needed to be calmer, more patient, and more reasonable in these hard times. And, for their part, that no matter how bad things get, looking at patients and their families through compassionate eyes can help improve communication and ease what is a searingly painful process. Hearing "we care about you" and "let us help you through this" could have made all the difference.

The doctors agreed to recommend that Harvey remain in the hospital for another day or two so that we had some time to find other accommodations. The hospital social worker brought me a list of nursing homes in the area that had openings—the same list I had been given when the doctor in the first rehab had told me to get a grip. Some had only one or two stars out of a possible five-star rating. Briefly I considered moving him back home with twenty-four-hour care, but that was even less a viable option than it had been when he moved out in May. He was much weaker, and we had already crossed that bridge. And the current fee of $22.50 per hour times twenty-four hours a day for in-home help was beyond comprehension—for an aide who would have nothing to do much of the time but who would require my help with transfers and medications around the clock.

I chose from the social worker's list a reputable skilled nursing facility that was close to our house. It was part of a hospital system we trusted. Our coverage allowed us to move Harvey there while I sought other alternatives. The next day, medics transported him to a real nursing home. He was only sixty-seven years old.

CRIES IN THE NIGHT

We entered a dark, windowless lobby, then passed through more doors leading to a nurses' station, in front of which seven or eight severely disabled elderly people were parked in wheelchairs. Some with oversized bibs were being fed; some were asleep; most were staring. Faded gowns and shapeless sweaters sloped across their slumping bodies. The inevitable bathroom smells assaulted us as we searched for our room number down the long hallway dotted with supply carts and people bent over walkers. My husband was wheeled into the back of a small room with a curtain divider, past a roommate who, we soon learned, had suffered the ravages of diabetes: he had lost his eyesight and both of his legs. His catheter had broken apart and foul-smelling urine had soaked his bedclothes. When he heard us coming in, he yelled out, "Miss! Miss! Would you hand me those potato chips on my tray?"

As we settled into a tiny space, I hoped, in my naiveté, that Harvey's debilitated physical condition would improve from the after-effects of infection and hospital confinement. Working with physical and occupational therapists, he would grow strong enough to be readmitted to the ALC.

How could I possibly have believed this?

The doctor at the nursing home was thorough, attentive, and kind as he pored over Harvey's copious medical records. Most of the harried nursing staff were doing their best to care for so many helpless patients. Unfortunately, Harvey had become so debilitated that the therapists could barely get him to stand. Once again, he was spending almost all of his time in bed.

Rooms for patients admitted for rehabilitation in this sprawling one-story facility were mixed with rooms for those under permanent long-term care. Although he had begun to look much older than his years, Harvey was twenty years younger than the average population. He was surrounded by women and men who had no idea where they were or who they were. Most had to be fed, medicated, diapered, and bathed in bed. Moans and cries echoed in the reeking corridors, where busy women and men wearing scrubs did their best to respond to so many needs. Harvey's roommate, who was completely helpless, with nothing to do, continued to holler at all hours. Tragically, in the weeks we were there, I observed only one visitor, one time—who said she was his wife.

Harvey's end of the room had no space for a visitor's chair, although not many visitors came. I submitted a request for him to be moved as soon as a private room became available. One afternoon, as I passed through the lobby, I saw a man using an upholstered chair as a toilet. I rushed to alert the administrative staff. The following day, the chair was still there, with some visible new stains.

On the first Sunday there, I set up my laptop computer on Harvey's rolling bed table so that he could worship with the live-streaming of our church service. I made sure he had his glasses and hearing aids, since the laptop sound was difficult to hear, and drew the privacy curtain. Then I left to sing in the choir. When I returned, the laptop was closed. Harvey said that his roommate had complained about the sound and Harvey, ever polite, had folded up the lid on the broadcast.

A few days later, he was moved to a curtained portion of another small semiprivate room, although without a roommate. One afternoon our senior minister came by for one of his much appreciated visits—he and Harvey always enjoyed their talks. I moved to the other side of the curtain to give them some time together. As I left, I heard Harvey asking him a question he had posed to me a few days earlier: "Is it all right to pray for yourself? I have always thought we should pray for others, but not ourselves." Then Harvey revealed that, throughout his illness, he had never once prayed for healing for himself. The minister assured Harvey that, indeed, God wants us to talk to him about our needs and concerns, including our own healing, our sorrows, whatever is on our hearts.

> *August 16, 2015*
> *Ann's Facebook Post*
>
> Watching church with the old man as he enjoys a hot Krispy Kreme donut. Thank you, Covenant Presbyterian Church, for live-streaming your services. It is such a wonderful ministry to those of us who can't make it in person. Hopefully this is Dad's last weekend here in the nursing home. In his words, he's had more transfers than Grand Central Station. #noideahowhecomesupwiththesethings
>
> Hopefully he'll be back at his apartment with his buddies early next week. Thanks for all your support!

As days stretched to weeks with little progress in therapy, Harvey was moved to a private room with a large window and extra chairs. I brought in birdseed for the feeders outside, but he was uncharacteristically disinterested in them. The very old lady next door, who wore a lacy white gown over her tiny bent frame, cried off and on throughout the days and nights. We could hear her calling, "Help! Help me!" When I reported this to the CNA on duty, she smiled sadly and said, "I know. We just changed and positioned her. She's done that for months—that's just what she does."

I asked, "But why does she have a feeding line?"

The nurse replied, "The daughter won't allow it to be taken out."

I thought about this for a long time as, on another long hall, a patient was screaming obscenities. I whipped around the corner to see several women in wheelchairs parked out in the hall. When I told the staff that the noise was disturbing other patients, they shrugged and gave me a look of helpless apology.

Meanwhile, Harvey was unable to make much progress in therapy, and the doctor added one more scary diagnosis: his lungs were filling with fluid, so he started regular breathing treatments with oxygen. He continued to lose weight. His Sweet's Syndrome had been causing odd rashes for years, but the newest manifestation was worst of all: slowly his body became covered with large hives and a smaller, fiery red rash that itched terribly.

As always, Harvey did not complain about his surroundings or his plight. He thanked each person who cared for him. He was patient. But he was disturbed by the wailing sounds echoing in the halls. He was in pain from his back and his rashes, and he was so very tired. He didn't want me to wheel him outside into the sunshine of the small garden. When I tried to set up a little picnic lunch for us there, he could hardly wait to get back inside to his bed. He groaned whenever a caregiver tried to get him to sit up. And he began having nightmares.

One night he called me about 3:00 a.m. "I am at Graham and Lisa's house and we are going out for lunch. Want to come?" I said, "I sure wish we could. But look around you. What do you see?"

After a few seconds, he replied, "Oh. I guess I'm not at Graham and Lisa's house."

Around that time, he made more strange calls to the children, his former co-workers, and others. One night he telephoned my sister in Durham and asked if they wanted to "join us for breakfast at the Sawmill," a restaurant four hours away in Wilmington. I could only hope that these hallucinations were caused by medications that could be adjusted.

At some point the ALC staff paid a visit to re-evaluate Harvey and, not surprisingly, again rejected his return to the facility. Even though we had continued to pay out-of-pocket for his room, it was evident that it was time to give it up. After an exchange of letters, the management agreed to refund a portion of our cash deposit and expenses for the time since Harvey left, as long as we vacated the premises by the end of the month. I was embarrassed at the way I had panicked when told Harvey was no longer qualified to live there, and I was resentful of the way they had handled his expulsion, and I couldn't make myself go back. The same loyal friends and the same movers who had helped us just two months earlier made the drive out, without me, to pack up and pick up Harvey's belongings. The new blue and green plaid bedspread, the comfortable brown lift chair, the nylon sweat pants and cotton tee shirts, his toiletries, his favorite plants, his stereo and books, all came back home in boxes and bags. The same moving company that had transported his few pieces of furniture out there brought it all back home. The following weekend, when I knew the regular staff would not be on duty and the place would be quiet, I drove out to pick up the last few items and turn in the key. I will never forget the kindness of the receptionist, aides, and fellow residents who spoke to me with concern and caring during those last minutes.

Meanwhile, a month into Harvey's stay at the nursing home, the social worker reminded us that Medicare did not cover nursing home fees unless a patient is in rehabilitation; in two weeks, Harvey would no longer qualify for rehab. He would then be considered a permanent resident, at a daily rate that would amount to thousands of dollars per month. *Oh, no,* I thought. *This place is not a good match for him. He is hallucinating and breaking out in hives here. He is miserable. He must move.*

But where could he go?

Chapter 14

Long-Term Care, Short-Term

All we can give back and all God wants from any of us is to humbly and proudly return the product that we have been given—which is ourselves.

Richard Rohr, *Falling Upward*

I began to research long-term care options in the area. Only one of the continuing care retirement communities (CCRCs) nearby accepted new residents directly into skilled nursing. Understandably, most reserved those rooms for their own residents who needed to transfer from independent living or assisted living. I even visited the facility in which Harvey's spry eighty-nine-year-old stepmother had settled into an apartment, but they had a long waiting list. Who would ever have imagined that his needs would grow to be greater than hers?

One morning, Graham and I toured two CCRCs. At the Presbyterian retirement home in which many of our fellow church members lived, we emerged from the car into the summer heat, surrounded by blooming roses, green lawns, and shrubs. I had visited there many times; Harvey and I had a number of friends already living there and others who had paid the deposit to add their names to the list for the future. But the only room available was a closet-sized cubicle at the end of a hallway between assisted living and skilled care, and Harvey would have to qualify for assisted living in order to be accepted. With little hope, I filled out the admission and financial forms and put down a deposit.

Next, we met with the admissions director of another CCRC that Harvey and I had toured two years earlier by invitation. To the sound of classical music, we strolled down its dark-green-carpeted hallways, past mahogany furniture, colorful paintings, fresh flowers, a library with a fireplace, a sparkling blue swimming pool, a cinema, a chapel, and a dining room with crisp white tablecloths and smelling of fresh herbs. We passed meeting rooms with easels announcing upcoming lectures on historical and local subjects of interest. We inspected the woodworking shop, pool tables, beauty salon, and the studio featuring oil and pastel paintings and sculptures by talented residents. We passed apartments that opened onto patios and manicured lawns. We could barely discern the transition from independent living to assisted living to skilled care. One hallway led to several well-appointed empty rooms for patients transitioning from one level of care to another.

But what difference would these amenities make for Harvey? Even if he could possibly be admitted there, would he ever be able to enjoy any of them? Since the most important factor for us was the level of personal care for patients, we were pleased to learn that the average length of employment for the staff was excellent.

I submitted application forms there, too. Then I met with our financial advisor to figure out how much more than our monthly income we would need in order to afford either place and where that money could come from. Medicare covers short-term skilled nursing care for rehabilitation but not long-term residential care. We had not planned to start liquidating assets this soon for retirement, but if we had to do it, we would. As always, I was keenly aware of how fortunate we were to have been able to save for retirement while paying premiums for a valuable disability policy. On examining the policy itself, I had discovered that long-term-care benefits would kick in the following year...if we needed them.

Nurses and social workers from both CCRCs would visit Harvey at the nursing home to observe him during therapy, assess his physical condition, and examine his medical records. Then they would notify us of their decision. Even though I knew he would fail to meet the requirements for assisted living, I alerted the head of the therapy department at the nursing home that observers were on the way. I remembered what the physical therapist from the hospital had told me during that phone call nine months earlier, and we were seeing exactly what she had meant by "end stage." It was more important than ever to find a safe, comfortable place for him to live with round-the-clock nursing care.

Less than a week before Medicare coverage ran out at the nursing home, Harvey was officially assessed by the CCRC staffs while the physical therapist patiently worked with him. As he sat in a wheelchair, she strapped a yellow gait belt around his waist. Then she helped him stand at the parallel bars. Weakly, he grasped at the right-side bar while she positioned his floppy left hand atop the other bar. Below his long gray athletic shorts, his bony, bruised legs and white running shoes began to shuffle forward. His thin white hair stuck up in all directions and his tortoise shell glasses slid partway down his nose as his bandaged arms drooped along the poles. His unshaven face was contorted in pain and determination; he understood the importance of this test. The observers were kind, their forced smiles betraying the pity and regret they felt. As I watched helplessly, I thought that I had never loved my husband more than in that moment.

Within days, the first response came. The Presbyterian home was truly sorry—they had so wanted to be able to approve our application. I could feel their compassion and desire to help. But Harvey was beyond assisted living status now. He had maximized his rehabilitation progress and needed permanent skilled nursing care, which was not available at that time to non-residents.

Now the only remaining choices were to stay at the nursing home or—please, please—to be accepted to the other CCRC. I was ready sell the house and do whatever I could to enable him to be cared for in a nice, quiet place for as long as he had left to live. Labor Day loomed, and it would be a long holiday weekend before we received the verdict. Feeling sick and shaky, I prayed they would call to let me know they had an appropriate space for Harvey.

Long-Term Care, Short-Term

Compassionate Encounters

While we waited for their decision, I received more bad news. But I also had encounters with two people who helped me to put our struggles into a broader context—to rise above complaint and focus more gratefully on signs of God's love in this world. These people were an appliance salesman and a minister.

The first encounter came as a result of a disaster report from our outside life. My sister telephoned from our Wilmington house, where she had planned to spend the holiday weekend. "I am so, so sorry to tell you this," she said, "but I just got to your house and it smells terrible. I opened the refrigerator and then I ran outside to throw up."

Sometime during the many weeks of our absence, a partial power failure from a defunct underground cable had worn out the refrigerator compressor, causing it to die and the small store of food inside to spoil. Jan discovered colonies of insects and mold inside it and black ooze seeping into the floorboards. A smaller refrigerator in the garage had died, too. I rushed to notify neighbors, hire a contractor, and file a claim with the insurance company. It would take months to repair the damage. But I couldn't be there in person to handle it.

Over that weekend, when I drove out to Sears to select a new refrigerator, I was assisted by a sales representative who was patient and kind. Obviously frazzled, I rushed him through the floor models while checking the specifications for my purchase with a neighbor by phone, explaining that I was in a hurry to get back to a sick husband. As he stood at the computer preparing my order, the saleman said that he was so sorry for my troubles. "It's hard, isn't it?" he empathized. I heard the sadness in his voice and looked up. "I had a son who was sick."

He used the word "had." Suddenly, I realized how self-centered I had been, feeling so sorry for myself that I had barely made eye contact. I looked this lovely human being in the face. "Your son?" I repeated.

"Yes," he responded, "he was getting ready to go to college. But he died of cancer last year." I hugged him, and I told him how sorry I was, and he hugged me back, and we both cried.

Later that day, I noticed that he had not entered his name on the sales slip in order to receive a commission. When I telephoned the store manager to correct the problem, I was able to commend my helper by name, adding, "You are very lucky to have him as an employee in your store."

The following day, another conversation also helped me to refocus. I sat in the heat outside the nursing home on a wooden bench to answer a call from one of the ministers of our church. I updated her on Harvey's situation and our dilemma. But what she heard beyond the desperation was the grief I felt in seeing my once vibrant husband so reduced, so debilitated—and my unwillingness to give up trying to help him get back to the way he was before the illness.

Here is what she said in response: "The essence of Harvey has always been his mind. His strength has always been his intellectual ability, his wit, his sharp mind. He still has that. So maybe now is the time to focus on those things. Not so much on his physical condition, but on who he really is."

Long-Term Care, Short-Term

I decided then to focus more on the essence of this man I had loved for so long. I would stop trying to push him to get better, stop chasing down therapists to discuss new ways to spur his improvement. Instead, I would enjoy the person he was. We would just be together. We would rest.

The day after Labor Day—just three days before the end of Harvey's approved stay at the nursing home—I received the call we had been waiting for: the CCRC had an open room in their transitional area; Harvey could move within forty-eight hours. Once again, I hired movers to transport a few pieces of furniture, a TV, and some belongings. I arranged his toiletries and set up bookshelves and pictures to make the room cozy, knowing he would be moved to another room in a week or two.

On September 12 at 12:42 a.m., after a nine-hour moving ordeal, I emailed our children to let them know their dad was settling into his ninth place in seven months.

"The PT folks have determined that Dad is too much for the aides to transfer so he has to be placed in a Hoyer lift every time he is moved. This is such a production that it won't happen often—he will be in bed almost all the time. He will be having meals in bed.

"Tonight a resident church friend came to the room and asked if I would like to eat with him in the dining room. While I was gone, Dad called me twice in fifteen minutes to beg for pain medication and ask when the Braves were playing. I just hope things will smooth out and we can find some peace and fulfillment. I know you all are super busy and have all kinds of stress in your own lives. I am sending this just

so we can all share in it as a family as we continue to need and appreciate your emotional support and love."

Thanks not only to the comfortable new surroundings but also to the new perspective I had been given, even with more medical emergencies to come, it seemed the day-to-day life that had been so frustrating over the past twenty-eight months had become more peaceful for what turned out to be the very short time we had left. Six days later, I fell and broke my collarbone.

The Breaking of Bones

On a Friday night in September, one week after moving Harvey to his newest temporary room, I met a friend for a late dinner. We shared a bottle of cold white wine. Then I went home and talked to both David, wishing him a happy birthday, and Ann. About midnight, I walked through the kitchen and slipped on a wet spot on the hardwood floor, landing at a hard angle on my left shoulder. It took me a long time, but I figured out that I could get up if I used my good right arm to immobilize my left arm. In the bedroom upstairs, I found that taking off my clothes was too painful, so, exhausted after a long and busy day, I lay down on the bed. A jagged bone was sticking up from the top of my shoulder just under the skin.

The next morning, driving with one arm, I arrived second in line at the orthopedic emergency clinic nearby. After taking a couple of x-rays, the physician assistant strode into the room and said, "Well, it's definitely broken."

Long-Term Care, Short-Term

"What's broken?" I asked.

"Your collarbone."

It was almost funny. Could there be a worse possible time for my first broken bone?

In fact, the clavicle had snapped completely, near the point at which it attaches to the shoulder. This was a tricky break that would require surgery to repair. I drove myself home with an immobilizing sling, a prescription for pain pills, instructions not to drive, a warning not to move much for fear of having the bone pierce the skin, and an appointment to see a surgeon on Monday morning. Before leaving the parking lot, I managed to text my friend with whom I'd had dinner the night before. She showed up at my house with a sheepish face and lunch; we had to laugh about the bottle of wine. A few hours later, after completing surgeries for the day, Graham arrived with a grandson and a box of warm Krispy Kreme doughnuts. Poor kids, I thought; once again, they are having to look after us. As expected, Ann offered to take days off from work to help me through surgery four days later that week.

I dreaded having to tell Harvey the news. When someone drove me to visit him that afternoon, his immediate reaction was, "I've been so afraid something like this was going to happen! You are hurt, and I'm not there to look after you!"

Septermber 19, 2015
Kandy's Facebook Post
  Thanks for all your encouragement and prayers. It seems our run of bad luck isn't over yet. I am having surgery on

> *Thursday to put my collarbone back in place. The break is in a bad spot that will require extra wiring. I will be in a sling for seven weeks before starting physical therapy for three months. The worst part is not being able to drive to see Harvey, who is doing okay at the CCRC. So the church is helping with an online calendar called Driving Miss Kandy. I will post a link later in the week in case you have time to help us out. Meanwhile, here is a word of wisdom for all: never walk across a wet spot on your kitchen floor, especially after having a little wine with your dinner.*

As word spread, friends began volunteering for duty. One took me shopping for oversized shirts that buttoned up the front and pants with elastic waistbands. They helped me dry my hair until I figured out a way to prop up the dryer on a towel rack and shake my head in front of it. They picked up clothes to be ironed and brought them back crisp on hangers. For the next month and a half, volunteers drove me to visit Harvey every day, prepared food, and purchased groceries and supplies for us. I hated feeling helpless and dependent, but I enjoyed their companionship. For days, Ann took care of my every need. I hated to add to her burden. On several of her many trips upstairs to see to my needs during the days after surgery, I saw the emotional pain on her face as she saw the physical pain on mine. But I simply could not have managed without her.

Long-Term Care, Short-Term

September 27, 2015
Kandy's Facebook Post

How to say goodbye and thank you to this precious daughter who took time off from work this week to take her mother to surgery, sat around the hospital for hours, handled the heavy ice machine for the hurting shoulder, held the barf bag, tramped up and down the stairs with food and drink, minded three dogs, changed sheets, did laundry, picked up and prepared meals, got the dead car battery recharged, and even cleaned out the pantry? Got up around the clock to administer meds, cleaned around the house, answered phone calls and texts, and still managed to be cheerful, funny, solicitous, and loving all the while? And all this following two and a half years of helping through the many crises with her dad? We are more than getting her back for her (fairly easy) childhood! This is love and blessing. Ann Cosper is the best.

October 7, 2015
From: Kandy
Subject: Calamity Cospers

Many of you already know our latest news, especially those following Ann Cosper's fun commentaries on Facebook, but I wanted to give an update to everyone. Since my latest email, Harvey has moved into his permanent room at the CCRC (address). He is getting PT and OT each five times a week toward the goal of growing strong enough to become more independently mobile. This means he is in bed a great deal of the time and is unable to take advantage of all the wonderful activities available there. He is working hard to get to the point that he is a "one person transfer" and can manipulate his own wheelchair (or, his goal: get back to using a cane someday). His energy and his spirits are often not very high, but he continues to be his usual kind and funny self with staff and visitors. He is getting good care and good food, reading a little, and following whatever sporting events are going on, including leading the Gridiron Geezers in the Cosper family fantasy football league.

Following a two-hour surgery for plates, screws, and wires, I am in a sling for a broken collarbone and unable to drive for six more weeks. Once again, we are overwhelmed at the kindness of folks offering help of all kinds. I just hope that, some day, I can be on the giving rather than the receiving end of human interaction.

For myself, I would appreciate your prayers for patience, endurance, and resistance to the temptation to cheat on my restrictions. For Harvey, we would appreciate your continuing prayers for hope, energy, improved health, and increased independence. He appreciates short visits (twenty minutes or so) between 3:00 and 7:30 p.m., and he does better with quiet conversation, as he is easily overwhelmed. That's all we need.

And just so you know, our luck hasn't changed yet. Assuming we must have run out of bad luck by now, a friend brought us two ten-dollar scratch-off lottery tickets

Long-Term Care, Short-Term

last week. He was going to split the millions with us. We didn't win a thing.

But we wake up every morning with healthy children and grandchildren, nice places to live (albeit apart), and the means to support ourselves, along with wonderful friends and our church family, and we are grateful for those.

UPS AND DOWNS, AND DOWNS

As I had since the first days following Harvey's stroke, I marveled at the people who rallied to help us. Not just the old friends but many whom we barely knew came to the rescue. Their assistance and companionship were invaluable during a time that both of us were incapacitated, and they taught me to accept help with more grace.

Harvey and I continued to enjoy books, word games, music, visitors, and following the Carolina Panthers' winning season. We enjoyed getting to know the staff, some of whom entertained us with stories about their lives in their home countries that we had never visited, including Liberia and Senegal, and we traced those places together on the big wall map in the hall. We filled out daily food orders for the trays delivered to his room, and the food service manager personally visited several times to make sure Harvey was receiving foods that he liked. Although he ate less and less, the enjoyment of food was one lifetime pleasure that served him well in those long days of illness.

Harvey perked up when I produced pen and paper to list his

favorite music. The activities director was starting the personalized iPod project, and Harvey was the first patient chosen for the experiment. For hours, he named songs, bands, symphonies, recording artists, and albums that he loved, from U2 to Chopin, from Chicago to Jimi Hendrix to Rodrigo's guitar pieces. He couldn't wait for me to show up in the mornings to tell me of additions to the list that he had thought of during the night. His knowledge of popular music was extensive. He remembered one-hit wonders and artists we hadn't thought of since the sixties. Thanks to a staff member and a volunteer at the facility, the iPod was finally delivered. I still have that list we made, and perhaps one day I will work on turning Dad's Greatest Hits into an eclectic series of recordings. I just wish we had thought to do this earlier, ourselves, so he would have had time to enjoy it.

There were many bright, interesting retired people living in the facility, and I tried escorting Harvey to a couple of events at which he could meet other residents: a lecture on World War Two and a luncheon for lawyers, for example. But sitting up had become too painful, and both times he soon asked me to wheel him back upstairs to bed.

Despite working with the personable therapists, Harvey continued to decline, so they started the process of tailoring a chair for him—either a power chair or wheelchair. A representative of the power chair company visited on several occasions. Harvey tended to run into things on the left side, including walls, furniture, and people. One day, he escaped in a trial scooter and lost his way in the labyrinth of hallways. After a frantic ten minutes with many of us searching for him, a fellow resident reported having spotted the fugitive in a different part of the building. We finally got him back to his room, and that was the end of the scooter trials.

Leaving the bed was so painful for Harvey, and moving him was so difficult, that we began to cancel outside appointments to the spine center, eye doctors, and the hearing center. Fortunately, the resident doctor at the facility was able to order tests and x-rays to be performed in the patient's room. He also referred Harvey to Palliative Care, a part of the excellent Hospice organization. A young social worker came to the room to explain that palliative care focuses on relieving the stress and pain of serious illness while treatment continues, whereas hospice care is prescribed to keep the patient as comfortable and pain-free as possible after treatment stops, when it is clear the person is not going to survive.

The long-awaited date for getting out of my sling turned out to be another day I will never forget. As shown by my posts that day, it proved to be another example of the ironies and stark contradictions with which we lived each day. When I walked triumphantly into Harvey's room to show off my freed arm, he was writhing in a wheelchair while suffering a seizure. It turned out to be a day in which, for the only time, a hospital failed to take care of us.

November 3, 2015
Kandy's Facebook Post

Hurray! No longer providing free advertising to Ortho-Carolina (though they have been great) with that giant black sling sporting their name in thick white letters—

even old ladies who break bones can heal! Can't lift anything over five pounds till after Christmas and have lots of physical therapy ahead. But how blessed are we who have the use of all of our limbs and who can be independent. And especially how blessed are we to have the love and constant support of our families, friends, and church community to get us through the hard times. Feeling grateful today!

November 3, 2015
Kandy's Facebook Post

So two hours after being cleared to drive, I used my newfound freedom to visit Harvey, who was having a major seizure, and then followed the ambulance to the hospital. The emergency department was full, so they left him on a stretcher in the hall for seven hours, surrounded by cursing, inebriated patients and gossiping employees, but they never did find out why the seizure occurred. He's safely back in his own room tonight for some well-deserved rest and TLC. His thirty years of defending the medical institutions didn't keep them from handing him a urinal to use on a stretcher in a busy public corridor. Fun day.

Two days later, I became ill from food poisoning. The day after that, I made a two-night trip to Durham for my niece's wedding. I was to host the bridesmaids' luncheon and sing during the ceremony, and Ann was a bridesmaid. It was impossible for

Harvey to make the trip—he could hardly sit up and rarely left the bed. It was difficult to leave him, knowing how much he wanted to be there with the family and how much he would be missed. My brother and his wife flew from Memphis to Charlotte to drive me to Durham in my car, since I was just finishing up my weeks in a sling. When we arrived, I had not eaten anything in two days.

I had advised everyone I could think of that I would be out of town. I furnished emergency contact information and devised a schedule of visitors for Harvey. As I practiced with the organist, entertained lovely young women and a beautiful bride, sang at the wedding, swayed to the songs of the band at the reception, visited with family, and slept in my modern hotel room, I envisioned my husband as he lay in his bed back in Charlotte. Was someone cutting up his food? Turning on his music? Responding to his call bell? Could he even find the call bell? Was he, in turn, imagining the family at the wedding without him?

I realized then, not just how much he needed me, but how much I needed him. I was relieved to get back to his side.

Chapter 15

Redefining Hope

"Let me light my lamp," says the star, "and never debate if it will help to remove the darkness."
Rabindranath Tagore, The Heart of God

How important is hope? How important is it that hope be based on practical reality, on what is actually possible or on what is most likely to happen? My hope throughout the preceding two-and-a-half years had been for Harvey to recover, or at least to improve toward a more independent life. But I had been blinded by hope not based in reality. Almost a year earlier, the therapist who called me had been right: my husband was not getting better. I had to find a broader definition of hope, a different kind of hope, identify something different to hope for. Because I didn't think I could live without any hope for him at all.

Harvey was failing—that was obvious. He was bed-bound. His muscles were wasting, and he was growing weaker. No one seemed to know why. His heart was bigger and floppier, but his lungs were now clear, and he did not seem to have any immediately life-threatening conditions. The worst symptom was the pain in his deteriorating back.

The Defense Rests

As Thanksgiving approached, I found myself hoping for him to continue living with as much comfort and dignity as possible. Hoping for him to find relief from pain and feel some joy and peace in each day. To continue being the grateful, accepting, and loving person he had always been. During the coming holidays, the family could see him together, and I expected he would be very happy about that. I didn't expect him to die.

November 21, 2015
From Kandy
Subject: re: Calamity Cospers
Latest update from the Calamity Cospers, a possible installment in a book full of disaster stories. We had another long day at the hospital yesterday: Harvey had outpatient surgery to repair a second compression fracture in his back. He had to be transported by stretcher with Medic both ways since he is unable to sit up (we tried wheelchair transport for pre-op visit Thursday, but delays forced him to be in the chair for five hours, as he was groaning and torturously slumped forward, unable to lift himself). Unfortunately, the medics weren't available to take him home until five hours after he was cleared to leave from the surgery. So he departed his room at 8:30 a.m. and did not get back until nearly 11:00 last night, having had nothing but clear liquids since the night before. Then, upon being fed some soup, he threw up.

We are praying the back pain will be eased once the surgery spot heals. He is already up for visitors.

My waiting-room boredom was interrupted by yet another distress call from Wilmington: the guy redoing the damaged floors following the power outage found rainwater seeping from the front porch into the doors and windows, all of which will have to be replaced before he can complete the job. And I haven't even been able to go down there in more than four months! Meanwhile, my physical therapist for my broken shoulder says she can't lead me in the proper exercises right now because I have tendinitis and nerve impingement.

However: our children and grandchildren and pets are all fine, and David comes home for a long visit one month from today. My sister and brother-in-law will join us for Thanksgiving and, though it will be so sad not having Harvey at the table with us, we will have fun going to see him. He'll probably be glad for the peace and quiet when we all leave. There are always many blessings to count, right?

The Cospers celebrated Thanksgiving dinner that year for the first time without "the old man" at the table. The grandchildren as always provided much fun and laughter. Afterwards, we took turns visiting Granddaddy in his room fifteen minutes away. It was hard to tell how he felt about his first Thanksgiving away from his family. He was glad to see everyone, interested in their lives as always, and sprinkling in his humorous observations. But as the day ended, everyone else went home and left Harvey alone in his room to sleep.

The Defense Rests

THANKSGIVING 2015
by Kathryn Cosper

The ghosts of Thanksgivings past
Hover and swarm in this big old house
Where I live alone now with the usual
Badly behaved wiener dog and a shaggy mutt
And the cardinals at the feeders—these are my family here now.
The laughing children and quirky parents,
the smell of roasting turkey filling the house
as we yawned down the stairs for juice and coffee
and people to tease and talk to;
Green beans snapping, gravy bubbling
As only their dad knew how to make it.
Always football—back yard and on television—
And a table of china with fall leaves and sparkling spoons,
Everyone talking and helping and eating and cleaning up
And talking some more, and laughing some more.
"What are you thankful for?" going around the table
from littlest to oldest, and "family" being the answer
Most often given. But this year…

The ghosts of Thanksgiving hover and lurk
In this big old house
where no one lives any more but me
and the two old dogs.
The little ones grew up and live other places,
Or have their own little ones and jobs and homes,
things to do and places to be.
They'll come around. New memories will grow.

Redefining Hope

But the founder of the feast—
ultimate roaster of turkeys and patient
maker of perfect gravy,
quipper of quips and lover of family,
struck even before old age with a clot
that went to his brain—
he lives across town
in his bed, and his chair with wheels, in a place
With nurses, where he won't fall any more.
Where are those old khaki shorts
And the dock shoes run down at the back?
Where are the celebratory drinks and toasts and the
Turkey baster and battered football and the
Comb-over we so lovingly made fun of?

The ghosts of Thanksgiving wander past
In this big old lonely house, where the porch he made
And the things he touched lie empty and still,
His suits lined up like old soldiers in the closet,
His side of the bed
Unwrinkled and cold.
People say you just need to find other things to be
thankful for—
And you do, of course.
But the ghosts of Thanksgivings past
Hover and die in this big old house
And fall around me like the dead brown leaves
Drifting and scattering in the chilly breeze of autumn.

The Defense Rests

Last Kiss

During the ensuing three weeks, Harvey's quality of life continued to decline. In the thirty-two months since the stroke, he had lost a total of seventy pounds. His pacemaker kept his heart rate from getting too low, but nothing worked in controlling atrial fibrillation, and his enlarged heart was increasingly less efficient. However, his mind was still good, his wit sharp, his compassion for others evident, and his faith strong. To the surprise of some of his caregivers, he continued to refuse to sign the bright yellow DNR form (Do Not Resuscitate); he had more living to do, he said, too many things to stick around for. Ann had met the love of her life, and he wanted to walk her down the aisle. He and the kids were going to visit all the baseball stadiums in the country. And there were so many fish left in the ocean off Masonboro Island.

In mid-December, after receiving reports of a little blood in Harvey's urine, the doctor ordered an x-ray that appeared to show a suspicious spot near his kidney. We panicked to think that he might, on top of everything else, have some kind of cancer. Harvey was once again scheduled for outpatient tests—this time a cystoscopy, which he greatly dreaded. He had to be put to sleep for the procedure. At 9:00 a.m. on Thursday, December 17, a wheelchair van transported Harvey to the hospital in a metal reclining chair. When admissions forms were being completed, once again Harvey declined to sign the DNR, saying, "I'm not ready for that yet."

The day turned out to be a mess of miscues and timing problems that made a suffering, disabled patient even more miserable. The hospital's inpatient rooms were full, creating a domino effect. Patients coming out of surgery were backed up in recovery rooms, so patients scheduled for surgery could not undergo their operations. With nothing to eat or drink since the night before, lying on a narrow stretcher, Harvey moaned in pain for hours in a cold, partitioned area. His five-minute procedure, scheduled for 3:00 p.m., was performed at 6:30 p.m. under general anesthesia. The urologist gave us the good news that, for once, no problem had been found; the blood was probably just the effects of blood thinners. By the time Harvey was awake and ready to leave the recovery room, it was too late for a transport back to his room at the CCRC. So he had to be admitted to a regular hospital room for the night.

The following day, after keeping our youngest grandchild for a few hours, I arrived at the hospital around lunchtime to find a cardiologist in the room. Harvey had developed a congestive cough, and once again his heart rate was erratic and high. A new medication had been ordered. Graham, as always, had been keeping up with the medical issues, visiting his dad and consulting with the specialists. The doctors agreed there was no reason for Harvey to remain in the hospital when he could be comfortably cared for back in his own bed with skilled nursing. His blood pressure was stable.

Around 4:00 in the afternoon, Graham helped us get organized and accompanied us to the familiar van parked in the circle in front of the hospital, where fountains were spraying lighted arcs of water into the air. As Harvey's reclining chair was strapped in, Graham leaned in and said, "I love you, Dad."

Today, when he has meetings in the hospital conference room overlooking the circle, Graham looks out the window and, in his mind, he still sees the van pulling away from the curb.

On our way back to the CCRC, Harvey looked out the window and remarked on how pretty the view was. His bed had been made up with clean white sheets and his room straightened, as usual. While he ate lasagna and drank sweet tea, I read aloud from a biography of Charles Lindbergh. We worked on some jumbles from the newspaper. We might have mentioned that our anniversary was the next day, and he might have quipped his usual, "We should all line up and get root canals in honor of the occasion."

Before heading home, I helped him get comfortable and positioned everything he might need within reach. He sounded congested. But he was propped comfortably in bed wearing his reading glasses, with the Carolina Wheels section of the paper open on his bed tray, hoping to find a Corvette to replace the one ("Granddaddy's blue race car") he wished he had not given up off the lease a couple of years earlier. Or maybe a truck. It didn't seem to matter to him that he couldn't even sit up by himself.

Cupping his stubbly cheeks in my hands, as always, I kissed him goodnight and asked if he had everything he needed. He said he was fine. We both said "love you" and, looking back from the doorway, I called out, "See you in the morning." It was 7:40 p.m. on December 18, 2015.

Part 4

When a Loved One Dies

Blessed are those who mourn, for they will be comforted.

Matthew 5:4

Do not be...terrified, for the Lord your God goes with you; he will never leave you nor forsake you.

Deuteronomy 31:6

In my father's house are many rooms; if it were not so, I would have told you. I am going there to prepare a place for you...I will come back and take you to be with me that you also may be where I am.

John 14:2-3

CHAPTER 16

MOURNING AND GRIEF

> *Sometimes our light goes out, but is blown again into instant flame by an encounter with another human being...Each of us has cause to think with deep gratitude of those who have lighted the flame within us.*
>
> Albert Schweitzer

YOU WEREN'T SUPPOSED TO DIE:
A LETTER TO HARVEY FROM KANDY

The first call awakened me at 2:42 a.m. Sounding breathless, the nurse said they were having trouble getting you to respond. She advised me not to leave home yet, because they might be sending you to the hospital. I jumped out of bed. What should I do? Where should I go? My breath caught in my chest and I began to shake as I pulled on jeans and a sweater. When she called again a few minutes later, I could hear someone counting out loud in the background. One...two...three... Chest compressions. The medics were there, she said. The heart kept stopping. Oh, my God! I told her I was coming. I called Graham. "Dad's in trouble." I made it to the car and started the short drive on the dark, foggy, empty streets. It was our forty-fifth wedding anniversary.

This couldn't be. It couldn't be happening. The doctors had cleared you to leave the hospital just a few hours ago. You had eaten supper. You were reading the paper. We were going to say "Happy Anniversary" tomorrow, and you were going to joke about root canals. You would have red roses delivered, as always. I would read to you and we'd laugh at our old family jokes. The kids would call. You were going to open your Christmas presents in a few days. You were going to hear about your big case being tried at the courthouse.

You were supposed to have a good retirement, with trips and fishing! We were supposed to get old and doddery together! You were supposed to dance at your children's weddings! You can't leave! Please don't go! God, please be with Harvey! Please! Don't let him die!

I found out later from the nurses on duty that, after I had left, you became increasingly uncomfortable, antsy, and anxious. You pressed the call button repeatedly, summoning them to your bedside, and they tried to comfort you. They took your vital signs, which weren't especially abnormal for you. You began talking to me, even though I was at home in bed and, Oh God! I couldn't hear you. You wanted to get up into your chair, but the nurses urged you to stay in bed—getting you up meant a miserable hoisting in the lift, pain for you and trouble for them. Then you said that you were cold.

They put warm socks on your feet. They wrapped you in blankets, like a cocoon. The nurse marveled in telling me that every time they responded to your call, you thanked them for coming, just as you always had.

Mourning and Grief

You called out, "Kandy, Kandy!"

"What did he say?" I pleaded. "What was he saying to me?" But she didn't know; she couldn't understand. "He sounded like he was giving instructions," she said—and you probably were. WHAT DID YOU WANT TO TELL ME?

You appeared to fall asleep, then you called out again. They wrapped you in another blanket and you seemed to doze off. They left the room. You stopped calling them. The next time they checked, you were not breathing. They called medics. They called me.

I was at a stoplight two blocks from you when she called to tell me they had stopped trying. You were gone. I had never before heard the sounds that came from me in the darkness that night.

Graham and I were kept in the hall for a while as the nursing assistants cleaned and prepared your body. When we were allowed to enter your room, you were still warm. You were dressed in a clean, light green hospital gown and covered to the chest with a thin cream-colored blanket. Your eyes were closed and your mouth slightly open. Sitting on the edge of the bed near your face, I tried to close it, but it slipped open again. You looked calm and peaceful. Your usually mottled skin was smooth and white. But not really like you. That body I had known and loved for most of my life, and yours, was there in the bed, those long bony feet with the toenails the kids always made fun of, the beautiful long hands that had touched and waved and loved and held, fixed the broken flywheel and lighted the grill, diapered our babies and raked our leaves and gripped the steering wheel and gestured before juries. I couldn't move from your side. I couldn't stop touching you lightly, your hands, your beloved face. I wanted to remember every single thing about you.

Graham was with us, with you and me. He touched my shoulders but I couldn't look back at him. How must he be feeling? I couldn't think of any way to help him. I couldn't think of much beyond your total stillness. You were gone. I wanted you to wake up. I was thankful for you, for your good life. I was overcome with love.

This couldn't be happening; it couldn't be real. The chaplain came to pray with us. Someone brought coffee on a tray. I think a couple of hours went by. It was like looking at a log fire, the way your eyes are drawn to the flames and you can't seem to look away. I didn't notice that the night staff had gathered, crying, out on the hall, until finally the funeral home men came to take you. They were waiting patiently down the hall.

I noticed your reading glasses on the table. We gathered up some plants and your little Christmas tree. I stopped in the doorway for one very last look. How could I leave? Forty-seven years of knowing you, and this was it. It was over. I would never see you again.

The Word Was "Great"

After we called David, Ann, Lisa, and Jan and Bob, Graham and I drove back to our house before the sun came up. He scrambled some eggs for us. I spoke with one of Harvey's sisters and with our senior minister, who scheduled a memorial service for Tuesday, December 22. We set an appointment for the funeral director to visit us in the afternoon. Then I sent out a brief email and Facebook post.

Mourning and Grief

About 9:30 a.m., a delivery truck pulled into the driveway. From the window, I saw the young driver step out with a vase of red roses. "Those are from Dad," I told Graham. "He must have asked Ann to order them for him." Graham met the fellow on the walkway and said, "My father just died a few hours ago, and those flowers are from him to my mother on their anniversary. I'll take them from here."

Bringing the roses into the house, Graham told me that, as the young man handed over the vase and turned to leave, he called out, "Have a GREAT day!"

We laughed and laughed. Harvey would have loved it. Cosper lore is full of flubs such as this one, and this was certainly one for the books. We would tell the story repeatedly. In fact, it's become a mantra: the following year on the anniversary of wedding and death, Graham would arrive at midday carrying a bag of sandwiches and an armful of red flowers with a card that read, "Have a GREAT day!"

The card Harvey had dictated for the flowers read, "Thanks for another great year, sweetheart. All my love, Harvey."

"Another great year," he had called it. I thought about the year we had lived through since the last anniversary—the hospitalizations, trauma, pain, moves, separation—all that he had suffered, all that he had given up, and Harvey was still grateful. He was still calling it "a great year." His last words to me were words of gratitude and love.

What he meant by that was so profound and yet so simple: to him, life was great because he appreciated all the good things. We had each other, and he was thanking me for being there with him and for him. Harvey had his family, his friends, and his immovable faith in God. For him, in spite of everything, it was a great year, a great life, because he believed he had everything that really mattered.

That moment reinforced to me not only a central truth about life, but also a truth about death: **loved ones who die continue to be present in our lives**. Even as I was entering a black hole of disbelief, numbness, loneliness, and sorrow, I knew that Harvey would be part of me forever. In stories, in laughter, in all the little and big ways, he was interwoven in who we were as individuals and as a family. From that moment, I wanted to immerse myself into everything about Harvey, the tangible and intangible. I wanted to talk about him, hear about him, and hug his friends.

Most of all, I wanted to share his gratitude. I wanted to focus on the good things, as he did. But I had a lot of work to do to get there.

December 19, 2015 7:25 a.m.
From: Kandy
Facebook Post and email

With the deepest grief imaginable, and also the deepest belief in the resurrection, I want to let you know that Harvey died during the night. While his heart rate was very high, he developed trouble breathing and lost consciousness. The staff was loving and attentive during efforts to revive him and in the hours that followed. A memorial service is planned for Tuesday at 11:00 at Covenant Presbyterian Church, with visitation following the service. I am so grateful for the blessing of forty-five years with this humble, gracious, funny, intelligent, and loving man and for the life of our family together.

December 19, 2015
Ann's Facebook Post

Today is my mom and dad's forty-fifth wedding anniversary. My dad died around 3:00 this morning. He had instructed me a few weeks ago to send her flowers today since he couldn't. The gorgeous roses arrived this morning with the card, which he dictated, "Thanks for another great year, sweetheart. All my love, Harvey."

I cannot imagine my life without him—my number one supporter, mentor, coach, personal hero, and the standard by which I measure a man's character. What a beautiful human being. I couldn't be more grateful for his life.

THE GIFT OF PRESENCE

What saved me was that I found gentle, loyal, hilarious companions, which is at the heart of meaning: maybe we don't find a lot of answers to life's tough questions, but if we find a few true friends, that's even better. They help you see who you truly are…help keep you company….

Anne Lamott, *Stitches*

There is a difference between mourning and grief. Mourning is the outward expression of grief, a necessary and unavoidable part of grieving. It includes actions and rituals. Grief is inward—the emotions, feelings, and thoughts experienced when we lose someone or something precious to us. We do both, but mourning seems to come first, whereas the real depths of grieving come after the crowds have gone home.

In the first hours and days following a death, there is so much to do that grieving takes a back seat to the ritual requirements of mourning. We have decisions to make: burial or cremation, funeral or memorial service or celebration, death notice or obituary. The house crowds with sympathetic visitors. Everyone needs something to eat and drink. Those from out of town need places to stay. The freezer fills with casseroles. We are looking for documents: the will, the insurance policies, the car title, details about personal history, and what was his favorite hymn? We have to file at the courthouse. Do we need a lawyer to help with settling the estate? We are going through the motions, in denial, numb. We get in our beds at night when the house is quiet and we are in shock. Has this really happened? We want to keep screaming, "No! You can't be gone. I just need to wake up. Come back!"

One of the first revelations I had about surviving the death of my loved one was that, **even though the hardest work of grief is done from within, the presence of loving family and friends supports, comforts, and inspires us to somehow find a way to keep going in a life that doesn't look like ours anymore.**

Within minutes after we began notifying our friends that Harvey had died during the night, messages began to come in by text, email, Facebook, the funeral home online site, cell phone, and land line. David was already en route for the holidays and was able to get home within a few hours. Ann and my sister arrived together. So many tears. So many hugs. So much disbelief. I was grateful for all the visits, messages, and floral gifts, as well. I knew there would be plenty of time in the days, weeks, and months ahead to be alone and quiet. Our bedrooms provided quieter space when we needed to mourn alone or in pairs.

For some people, being surrounded immediately by others is difficult, if not intrusive. I've heard people say, "Give the family time to grieve." But it's up to each individual in each family to make that call personally, and it's up to friends and acquaintances to discern and honor it. Sometime later, one of Harvey's closest friends and associates told me, "Two of us came by the house that afternoon, but it was obvious that David was just getting home from the airport, and we didn't come in." That was respectful and kind. If the family—or someone in the family—is grieving privately and not receiving guests, even days or weeks later, we must not be offended. We can understand that the visit was not wasted; the fact that we cared enough to be present is appreciated.

For me, in those first days it was comforting having people around. They loved him, too, and it was good to hear that affirmed, to talk about him and tell stories, to share the grief in community. But I was also numb and disbelieving, going through the motions. The hardest times would be when my numbness wore off and reality set in, over the weeks ahead.

Throughout the day, friends streamed up the front steps with ham, sandwich platters, salads, desserts, drinks, and snacks, along with hugs and tears. Flowers and plants filled the house with color and perfume. The Covenant Bereavement Committee delivered a tub of paper towels, napkins, cups, and other helpful items, and they offered a meal for the family. They were also sending someone to take care of the house during the memorial service to answer calls and deliveries and to make sure the home was safe.

I was being pulled in many directions. I needed **someone to take charge of the activities at home**—and someone did: my sister started **a list of all the calls, visitors, food and other gifts that were brought or delivered, including descriptions and/or photos of flowers whenever possible.**

Practical help to make the house ready for company is invaluable. Mid-morning, Graham was sweeping the front walk when a neighborhood couple who were long-time friends asked him for the broom, saying, "Let us do that. You go and do something else that you need to do." A few minutes later, they stood at the front door in their old jeans and, after hugs of sympathy, asked me, "Where is your toilet brush?" Knowing the house would soon be overflowing with family and guests, they proceeded to clean. Here was a new humorous storyline Harvey would have loved: on her next birthday, I delivered to them a new toilet brush adorned with a big white bow. And when I learned that the beloved husband of a friend had died a few months later, I drove to her house to look for the broom and started sweeping. It was such a terrible broom that I later bought her a new one, tied a white bow around it, and left it on her porch.

Offering photos and mementos is a good way to honor the loved one. One friend took our family's Christmas photo cards from

Mourning and Grief

past years and created "Cosper Christmas" posters. We displayed these at the memorial service, and they continue to decorate our home every Christmas. Since Harvey had expressed concern that his grandchildren would not remember him as healthy and whole, I later preserved memories of him with printed book of **pictures and stories** from his life – a book entitled "Granddaddy was a Very Big Man," with short narrative and many photographs.

We might not think it means much just to sit in the pews, but families do appreciate our **attending the funeral or memorial service**. I was certainly grateful that people made the effort to be there with us on that raw December day, and many waited in a long line to speak to us personally. I sometimes return to the registry they signed at the church and feel glad for their presence with us to honor Harvey. Since then, I have made a greater effort to attend funerals of people I know, or whose families I know. I also make a point of **sitting closer to the family** than I would have before, as my Bible study group and best friends did for me. That way, instead of being isolated, the family will feel as surrounded by love as I did at the worst time in my life.

The important thing is not to ask what we can do, because the family is overwhelmed and has no idea what needs to be done, but to think of something we can do to help… and just do it. A minister of pastoral care at our church used to say that the most important words following a death are "I came as soon as I heard." **Whether we bring breakfast foods, sweep the porch, order flowers, purchase a special handkerchief, collect pictures of better times, share memories, or just drop by for a hug, we can provide the gift of presence.**

The Defense Rests

FIRST WRITTEN RESPONSES TO THE FAMILY

Email and text messages provide easy avenues for timely response when we wish to share right away in the grief of a friend. Family members will need time to share their own news first; then, a responding message is appropriate. There is an important difference between a Facebook post, for instance, and a message or comment in response to a post by someone else. We share others' personal news only with their permission. We were comforted by the many messages of love and support we received.

Personal sentiments such as those in the examples below, and in the next chapter on sympathy notes, mean much more than the overused "you are in my thoughts and prayers" and "I am sorry for your loss." It's so much more than a "loss," as though we are talking about the stock market. Such meaningful responses are ways to **enter other people's grief with compassion and love, bringing tears and laughter, refreshing memories, engendering gratitude, and helping them find the strength to get through the day.**

- "Today I learned that my dear friend Ann lost her precious father Harvey after a long struggle with poor health on the day that her mother Kandy had hoped to celebrate their wedding anniversary. He was a warm, witty, and wonderful man whom I adored fiercely. I have had the sincere honor of having witnessed the unconditional and powerful love he had for his family, his enduring faith in times of immeasurable challenges, and his unparalleled humor when there was nothing left to do but laugh at

the hand that life had dealt to him. Harvey… it's a small comfort to know that now you're looking down… and watching over us with your loving grace and goodness."
- "Today is a very sad day for me. One of the best men I've ever known passed away last night. He was kind beyond measure and humble to a fault. He was funny (he reveled in puns) and he was an incredible father to my best friend. From the first time I came over to their house over twenty years ago, he treated me like one of his own. Think of all those new people he has to tell all his classic jokes to up in heaven."
- "Ann, my heart aches for you and your family. I've thought of you all day wishing I had words to soothe some of what I can't imagine you and your family are experiencing. I didn't know your dad, but wish I had. His character as portrayed through your Facebook posts always warmed my heart and put a smile on my face."
- "I cannot put into words my sadness. I am so grateful I got to know Harvey through you. May God surround you and your family with his peace and grace! I am in awe of your love and constant care for Harvey."
- "Harvey is missed today. I have a big empty feeling."
- "Dearest Kandy, My heart is so very heavy for you and your family today. There are really no words that will offer much comfort at the moment, I'm sure, but please know that there are so many out there today and for so many days into the future who are thinking of you, aching for you and will be doing for you what we can to help through this most difficult time."

- "I doubt you can recall all the faces of those who knew you and Ghost (as we called Harvey in our Chapel Hill days). I would like to thank you, and in absentia Harvey, for the wonderful camaraderie we experienced in the fraternity. You set a wonderful example of how we can be brought together in a bond of friendship by principle quite independent of both religious and political dogma that so clouds so many of our lives today. It was truly gratifying to hear that you and Harvey had managed to stay married for so long. Thank you for all you are and all you have been to so many others."
- (from a widow of a young lawyer) "This is a note to let you know that we join with so many in thinking of your family here at Christmas and in all times to come. It is also to let you know that you can do this next stretch of days with your characteristic strength, pluck, and tremendous grace... *You can do this hard thing.* And Kandy, it doesn't have to look a certain way. You do not have to say, feel or be a certain way. You can do this hard thing one step, one breath, one moment at a time. You are strong. You are brave and God is present always. We love you, wonderful, indomitable Kandy. Hang in there."

COLLEAGUES ARE MOURNING, TOO

It's important to acknowledge that **not only family members but also colleagues and friends grieve** for those they have lost.

Mourning and Grief

Here are a few examples of expressions of sympathy that were sent to Harvey's co-workers at the law firm. They comforted his friends and expanded my vision of his life outside the home. I was grateful that they shared these with me.

- "Harvey was my law school classmate and has been a wonderful friend ever since. I have never known an attorney who was so gentle yet so effective. He was loved by all who knew him. We have lost a giant among us who can never be replaced nor forgotten. Rest in peace, my friend. Well done, good and faithful servant."
- "An extraordinary advocate, honorable soul and dignified human being. Harvey's caliber would be difficult to match."
- "Harvey was truly one of a kind. He was a fierce advocate for his clients and what was right and just. But even more importantly, he was as kind and fine a gentleman as any of us has ever known. He will be missed."
- "I know you are all mourning the loss of a great mentor and friend. There are no words that can express how I personally feel about Harvey and what an influence he had on me as a young lawyer. He is and was everything good about our profession. What a great man who will be greatly missed by all."
- "Such sad news. Harvey was one of the best in every respect."
- "Sincere condolences to Harvey's family and colleagues. He was such a fine example, professionally and otherwise."
- "Harvey was our Atticus."
- "Harvey was a great lawyer and an even better person. He

will be sorely missed."
- "He will be terribly missed by all who knew him, but his reputation will be honored for many years to come. I tried my first case with Harvey. If this were a typical senior partner/young associate story, my 'trying' the case with him would have amounted to my more or less carrying his bag and doing the behind-the-scenes work while he got to do all the exciting, 'front stage' work. But lucky for me, that wasn't how Harvey did things. Not by a long shot. We shared the front stage work— and the back stage work. When I showed up to the office to prepare for trial on Saturday mornings or late at night, I would arrive to find him already there, surrounded by papers and planning for whatever was to come next."
- "Harvey was a gentleman of the highest order. All who knew Harvey had the greatest respect for his talents and generosity. Rest in peace, Harvey. You will continue to be missed."

Rituals of remembrance and celebration

Writing an obituary and planning a funeral or memorial service can be comforting ways to express grief, share memories, honor the person who died, and give perspective on the loved one's life.

When the funeral director arrived, we learned that we had less than an hour to submit an obituary in order to have it published in the Sunday edition of the *Charlotte Observer*. So the family sat in the den together, my hands flying over my laptop keyboard, and composed words that would surely not do justice to the life of this man we had loved and who had loved us so well. It was difficult to write because Harvey was so humble; he would have been happy with a two-sentence announcement. But it was also easy to write because the story of his life, and the picture of who he was, poured out of us through both tears and laughter. As we reminisced that day, and over all the days since, we have found ourselves crying one minute and laughing the next. These disparate spirits continued when Lisa arrived with a family favorite, her homemade lasagna, along with the three grandchildren, who folded themselves into my arms and said, "I'm so sorry Granddaddy died."

It comforted all of us to know that Harvey was with the God who had loved and walked with him throughout his life. We imagined all the things he could be doing in heaven, now that he was whole and healthy again, and we knew that, wherever and whatever heaven was, it was a place of even more kindness and fun because he was there, with the people he loved who had arrived before him.

I modeled for the family a black sleeveless dress with three different jackets that I could add: powder blue, royal blue, and red. Everyone either expressed an opinion or said to "wear whichever one you are most comfortable with." Would anyone think it inappropriate to wear red to her husband's funeral, I wondered? But then someone asked, "Which one would Harvey like the best?" I thought of the red roses, and the unimportant decision was made.

Three days before Christmas, people filled the beautiful sanctuary of our church for a Celebration of the Resurrection for Harvey. The service was live-streamed on the internet for friends and family who were unable to attend. Rows of church elders processed to the front pews in honor of Harvey's service as one of them. As the family filed in across the aisle, I caught a glimpse of my long-time Bible study group and close friends sitting in the rows right behind us. So often, people attending funerals leave empty rows behind the family. My friends enclosed us in a strong expression of love and solidarity. I settled into the dreaded seat of sorrow in the front pew where I had seen so many widows and other sorrowful people sitting over the years. Now it was our turn, and I could hardly believe it was real.

We chose as the opening hymn "Joy to the World," and I had to smile as I heard Harvey's deep bass on his favorite "heba-nebba-nature sing" refrain. The choir sang "Set Me as a Seal Upon Your Heart." We all sang "For All the Saints" and Harvey's favorite hymn: "The church's one foundation is Jesus Christ her Lord. She is his new creation of water and the word...." It ends, "Lord give us grace that we, like them the meek and lowly, may live eternally."

Our minister professed that he had an onerous task for two reasons: first, in speaking before so many lawyers and judges in the crowd; and second, because the person whom we had gathered to celebrate would never want to be the center of attention. In that context, he spoke eloquently about Harvey through the reading of scripture while making God the center of attention. The prophet Micah's admonition to "do justice, love kindness, and walk humbly with your God"—the message on Harvey's retirement gift and hanging on his wall—was the central message of his memorial service. I glanced at my littlest grandson sitting quietly in his father's lap beside me; at the two older grandchildren; at Graham and Lisa, at David and Ann on either side of me. What must they have been thinking and feeling? I prayed that all of us would always remember these words in living our own lives.

After Widor's "Toccata" from *Symphony no. 5* rang out from the organ, we visited with people who waited in a line that stretched from one building to the next on that cold, misty day. The beautiful arrangements of red and white flowers from the sanctuary were moved to the center of the buffet table that offered a light lunch. The red roses Harvey had sent for our anniversary centered a table of photos from his life. As family and significant others supported us from the side, the children and I greeted many loving friends, hearing many kind comments and good stories. It was hard to talk about Harvey without smiling and chuckling. One friend got right to the point: "Harvey is up there right now laughing about how many billable hours are going to waste with all these lawyers here today."

December 22, 2015
Ann's Facebook Post
  I could not be more overwhelmed or more grateful for everyone who attended Dad's memorial service today, or attended online, or has texted me or messaged me or called me. It means the world to see how many lives my

dad's life touched. He was an incredible lawyer but an even better human being and father. This still feels like a dream from which I'm praying to wake up. I wish I could tag everyone who has reached out, but Facebook limits the number of people you can mention. Each of you has left a mark on my heart. Thank you, thank you, thank you. I love all of you and I thank God for each of you in my life.

December 24, 2015
Ann's Facebook Post

Lying in bed in my childhood room in the dark listening to the rain and wondering how life continues without the one I held most dear. This is where he taught me to say my prayers, where he carried me and laid me down after I had fallen asleep elsewhere in the house. Where he read me books and told me stories and woke me up for church and school. He delighted in me and I in him. There was no safer place in the world than in his arms. Whenever I came down the stairs to go somewhere, he told me I looked great. He believed in me when I didn't believe in myself, and in every dream I ever had, and he did everything he could to make all of them come true. He quizzed me on school topics and helped me become a better athlete. We had comfortable silence standing by the grill in the cool evenings enjoying each other's presence. There will never be another hug like those from him. And there will not be a similar joy that I had as a little girl when I heard his car pull into the garage or the sound of *his hard-soled shoes when he came home from work. He was my hero and I thought he was the greatest man I had ever known. And he is and I do and I always, always will.*

Eight Practical Tasks Following Death of a Family Member

1. After doctor or coroner has signed certificate of death, contact funeral or crematorium director. You will need at least ten copies of the certified death certificate, which will be required by insurance companies, banks, and other accounts listed in the deceased's name (e.g., utilities and credit cards). Funeral directors often will handle this for you.

2. List people to be notified: clergy, relatives, friends, employers, insurance agents, Social Security, and family or estate attorney, if applicable. Coordinate phone and social media notifications. Consider plans to accommodate guests from out of town.

3. Accept help preparing living area, kitchen, and bathroom for guests and for recording visitors, callers, food, flowers (photos are helpful), and gifts. Funeral directors can provide notebooks for these records as well as printed acknowledgment cards.

4. If you have kept a file of vital information in the event of death, or made plans in advance with a church or funeral

service, your job will be much easier. (See Chapter 2.) Create a file including the deceased person's date and place of birth, parents (birth certificate, if available), family members with contact information, CV, photo, and other information for death notice or obituary. Most newspapers charge by the line and have strict submission deadlines.

5. For funeral or memorial service, meet with officiant. Decide on place and time, music, flowers, transportation, participants, clothing, reception venue and food, if desired, and any family pictures or other memorabilia you might want to display.

6. Locate the will, powers of attorney, and marriage certificate, if applicable. Identify assets owned jointly and those owned solely by the deceased. The county requires an estate accounting of assets and debts in the deceased's name. Take documents, along with death certificate, to the county courthouse. The clerk will provide forms to return by a required date. An estate attorney can be invaluable, completing forms, meeting filing requirements, and handling many other duties during a time of stress. Simplified probate might be available.

7. Before notifying the bank of the death, check on access to joint accounts ("right of survivorship") and online bill-pay options once they receive the official death certificate.

8. Deliver copy of death certificate to a local newspaper for the legally required public notice of death to possible creditors.

CHAPTER 17

Words for Expressing Sympathy

Our culture treats grief like a problem to be solved or an illness to be healed. We've done everything we can to avoid, ignore, or transform grief. So that now, when you're faced with tragedy, you usually find that you're no longer surrounded by people — you're surrounded by platitudes...

The last thing a person devastated by grief needs is advice. Their world has been shattered. Inviting someone — anyone — into their world is an act of great risk. To try to fix, rationalize, or wash away their pain only deepens their terror. Instead, the most powerful thing you can do is acknowledge. To literally say the words: I acknowledge your pain. I'm here with you.

Note that I said with you, not for you. For that implies that you're going to do something. That's not for you to enact. But to stand with your loved one, to suffer with them, to do everything but something is incredibly powerful.

Tim Lawrence,
"The Adversity Within: Shining Light in Dark Places," blog

When we lose someone we love, **nothing anyone says or does can make the pain go away.** It will be there always, its intensity rising and falling over time as a constant companion. Grieving people appreciate, even need, expressions of caring and love. Just the fact that others care enough to take the time to **comfort the family with visits, calls, cards and letters** means a great deal. Some expressions of sympathy, however, are more welcomed than others.

Words that are Not Helpful after a Death

As I have been informally surveying people to find out the "best and worst" things others said to them during times of illness and death, I have heard strong agreement in their responses, particularly to the question of what not to say after a death.

- **"I know how you feel" is the most commonly unappreciated response.** As discussed in Chapter 3, this well-meaning attempt to share feelings minimizes the experience of the suffering person. It is important that we be present with our bereaved friends in their situations and not make our conversation about ourselves. It's best not to tell our "death stories" until later, if at all.

    In "We Need to Talk: How to Have Conversations That Matter," author and talk show host Celeste Headlee described an encounter she had with a friend who was grieving over the death of her father. Headlee started telling her friend how her own father had died when she

Words for Expressing Sympathy

was very young, saying, "At least you had your father in your life longer than I did," and concluding with "I know how you feel." The friend responded, "No, you don't know how I feel," and left abruptly in tears. The author said:

"When I began to pay a little more attention to how people responded to my attempts to empathize, I realized the effect of sharing my experiences was never as I intended. What all of these people needed was for me to hear them and acknowledge what they were going through. Instead, I forced them to listen to me and acknowledge me."

The truth is that each of us is unique. The only person who knows how you feel is you, and sometimes you don't know yourself.

- **Bereaved people do not want to be told "You must be relieved" or "It was a blessing."** In fact, they don't want to be told how they must feel. Many grieving people have expressed their frustration at hearing these comments from others. "Are you serious?" they want to respond. "My wife is gone! After a long life together, I will never see her again. No—I am not relieved." One of my closest friends cared for a sick husband for many years. The last seven months of his life, he never moved from a hospital bed in their den. With help for just a few hours a week, she turned him every two hours around the clock and took care of his every need. He was near the point of death for days before his breathing finally stopped. Yet she felt angry to the point of tears when people said after he died, "It must be a relief." Another friend who cared for his wife during seven years of Alzheimer's disease said he did feel a sense of release for her. But his beloved wife was gone and, in the finality of it, he grieved deeply.

Surely, living with illness can become so painful that letting go can be seen as a relief. Some grieving people do feel this way. But **it is up to those who mourn, not other people, to put their feelings into words.** Bereaved persons might already feel guilty and selfish for wishing their loved ones were still alive in spite of their illness and misery, for not feeling relieved. Others might feel guilty and selfish for being relieved. **We cannot change how they feel; we can only honor it.**

- **Grieving people may not want to hear that the person who died is "out of their misery" or "in a better place" or "finally at peace."** And, as explained in Chapter 3, **it's best not to suggest that "everything happens for a reason" or "time will heal" or "this is the will of God" or that "God needed another angel."** Does God cause people's loved ones to die in order to furnish himself with companions? If any of those statements make them feel better, they've already had those thoughts themselves.

The person who has died is not just the person who was sick at the end. For me, I was missing not just Harvey as he was, weakened and frail, at the end of his life, but the whole person I knew for nearly fifty years. The lanky student in the oxford-cloth shirt with whom I fell in love at Carolina, the man who held our babies in his arms and kissed them, the father who cried at his son's wedding and his own father's deathbed. Who worked so hard to provide his family with a secure and stable home. The guy in the khaki shorts firing up the grill on Saturday night and throwing the baseball with the kids in the back yard, the husband who reached for me at night and stayed by my side throughout a good life together with humor, grace, and love.

The point is that, even if the last months or years of a person's life are full of pain, that person was also once lively and vibrant, and it's the whole person that we miss. Whether it be my lifetime partner, the mother and father who raised me, the child I raised, the friend who shared life's biggest moments—no matter the circumstances of death or the years of struggle, no matter whether the death was sudden or drawn out for years—we are sad beyond words, and we will miss them always.

- **Anything starting with "at least" is not comforting or helpful.** As much as we would like to make sad people feel better, there is nothing we can say to friends who are mourning to talk them out of their anguish. They already have, within themselves, the beliefs, comforts, and insights that are uniquely their own. It doesn't help when others try to force them to find a bright side to the death of a loved one. I have heard of shockingly insensitive attempts to do so, as though human beings are interchangeable or replaceable: "At least you are young and you can marry again," "At least you have other children," "At least you can have another baby."

When comforting a friend at the time of a death, we can rarely go wrong by saying we are sorry and by saying good things about the person who has died. ("Passed away" is a euphemism that some people like. I personally never use it.)

- **Unless they specifically ask for it, grieving people are not looking for advice—not on how to handle the funeral, what their immediate plans for the future should be, what they should be doing, or how to feel better.** It's best not to ask the survivors whether they will sell the house, spend more time someplace else, go back to work, take up a hobby, or any such future plans. **It is important to respect their personal choices and allow them to grieve in their own unique ways.** No matter what decisions they eventually make for the future, their lives will never be the same. And the journey of grief will last a lifetime.

  The exception to this may be with a friend who continues to languish in grief, unable or unwilling to leave the house or engage in any social activities for many months. When this happens, close friends might want to carefully and lovingly engage the person in conversation about possible ways to ease back into a more normal daily life.

- Finally, we want to be careful about asking for personal details, like **"What happened?"** or **"How did she die?"** or **"Were you with him?"** Instead, we can take the conversational lead from the grieving person, who might or might not want to talk about the cause and manner of death. We especially want to avoid questions that seem to cast judgment—for example, "Was he alone when he died?" "Had she seen a doctor about it?" "Did she smoke?" or, following a car crash, "Was he the driver?"

Words of Comfort and Remembrance

Suggestions for what to say to a grieving person are much the same as those described earlier for illness. The most heartfelt sentiments can be conveyed in the simplest words:

- **I am so sorry.**
- **There are no words to express my sadness.**
- **So many people loved and will miss…**
- **I love you. I care about you. I am here with you.**
- **So many of us are grieving with you right now.**
- **I have such wonderful memories…I will never forget…**
- **I am here if you want to talk about it.**

Most grieving people I have known do want to talk about the death, whether right afterward or sometime later; some of us tell the story over and over again. These conversations are difficult for the listener, who might not know how best to respond. Bereaved people often blame themselves or others, including medical providers. There is not much we can say except to follow the rules of listening with responses such as **"This is so hard," "It doesn't seem to make sense right now,"** and **"I know you'll** need time to think and process it all. Meanwhile, I am here with you every step of the way."

Grieving people like to tell and hear **personal stories and positive comments** about those whom they have lost. On a deeper level, these sentiments help a mourner to reinforce gratitude for the life of the person who has died and the relationship they enjoyed together.

The best responses are uniquely personal. Even when we send purchased pre-printed cards, it is important to sign them with personalized messages. These sentiments help grieving families to

- **expand their vision beyond the illness and deathbed to their wider life together,**
- **confirm the qualities that made the loved one who she or he was,**
- **build stories about the impact they had on other people,**
- **confirm when the family experienced a life of love together, and**
- **acknowledge the depth of their grief.**

When we are writing to a bereaved person, even if we did not know the loved one who died, we can personalize the message. For example: "I wish I had known your mother. From your stories, I can tell she was a lively and funny person who brought joy to others. She must have been so proud of you and your children."

Again, instead of offering a one-size-fits-all suggestion of how to write a meaningful sympathy note, I have selected a sampling from the kind letters and cards we received in the weeks after Harvey died. I include the following as examples of personalized messages from people who knew us in different ways, not to immortalize Harvey or to set him up as special—although, if you come away thinking so, that is perfectly fine with me.

From People Who Knew Him But Not Me
The following card, signed by a husband and wife I never knew, was one of the most meaningful that I received. It was postmarked the day after the obituary appeared in the newspaper, addressed to my real name of Kathryn and sent in care of our church.

"Kathryn, Harvey was a kind, caring person and it was always a pleasure, when he came to the Coffee Shop, seeing him. May wonderful memories always keep you and your family smiling. I'm smiling now."

Signed by the owners of the coffee shop in the Law Building.

From the Therapist Who Had Called About "End Stage"
Another unexpected note arrived from the physical therapist who had called a year earlier to help me understand that Harvey was not going to get better. I quote it here in its entirety:

"After reading Mr. Cosper's obituary I wanted to reach out to you and thank you for bringing him by the clinic in the fall to see me. It was such a surprise and something I will always cherish as that took thoughtfulness and genuine kindness. As a therapist I work diligently to restore my clients' health to their former abilities. Unfortunately, I often find myself working to help folks embrace a new normal and this is never easy. I spend time praying each morning for my clients and their families and asking God to let His hands help mine. I regret I couldn't get Mr.

Cosper back to his boat, something he talked about. He seemed more at ease with his challenges than I did, and his gentleness and wisdom blessed my life.

"Kandy, thank you for pushing Mr. Cosper to recover his maximum. I believe it is very difficult to be a caregiver, especially as the spouse as there's a fine line between being an encourager and an irritation. There's also sleep deprivation and energy expenditure to recover. There's worry, planning, decision-making and loss. Kandy, please know I hope 2016 will afford you restoration, readjustment and reformation. I care about you too. That's something Mr. Cosper would have respected deeply, I think.

"May God divinely bless you and your family during this transition and give you the sustenance required to continue this journey along a new path."

FROM A FRATERNITY BROTHER WE HADN'T SEEN IN YEARS
"I am sorry to hear of the passing of 'the Ghost.' I never heard of anyone who didn't love and respect him. He was always someone who was pleasant and enjoyable to be around and a stand-up guy who you were proud to say was your friend. Obviously, he attained a great deal during his life and did it the right way which these days is very rare. Many will miss him including me. With deepest sympathy..."

FROM A DOCTOR WHOM HARVEY REPRESENTED
"I am so sorry about Harvey's passing. There is no finer man that has walked this earth. He is the perfect role model for any man to emulate, filled with integrity and compassion. I loved

reading about him today and the story captured him perfectly. I will never forget and always appreciate what he did for me (a sentence I know you will read many times in the days to come). We were all blessed to know him. Love…"

FROM AN OLD FRIEND (BEST PRE-PRINTED CARD)
In the Loss of Your Husband
I believe in my heart of hearts that extra love and grace are being sent to you.

I believe that your husband's presence will be there to support you through the years to come in ways you cannot yet know.

And I believe in you – your amazing, loving heart will find a way to carry on and smile again.

And signed, "Harvey was the kindest, most wonderful man I ever met. I know you miss him so much."

FROM A YOUNGER CO-WORKER
"Harvey didn't just 'practice law.' He embodied everything we all wish we could be. He is what we all imagined when we filled out our law school applications. The pure honesty coupled with knowledge and a profound appreciation for justice is what we all believe a lawyer should be.

"Thank you for sharing Harvey with all of us. The world is a better place because he was in it. I wish I had done a better job of thanking him.

"You two were a perfect partnership, relationship and marriage. I have difficulty thinking of any other couple consistently displaying profound respect and appreciation for each other. For all of us on the outside looking in, the Cosper family was about as fine a family as you could imagine. I know he will be terribly missed. I pray you and your family will find peace. I know it will never be the same without him; but it seems like that's what we are all supposed to say.

"You know all this already, but I just hope it is something to hear one more voice in support of the kind, brilliant, gentle and sincere man you married."

FROM AN OLD FRIEND
"Whenever I was with Harvey throughout the twenty-eight years we knew each other, I always did feel calmness in his presence and I always smiled."

FROM A FELLOW CHURCH MEMBER
"My dear Kandy, I've waited so long to write because the loss you and your family have experienced is so profound as to be intimidating. I was afraid of writing something not only inadequate but just dumb. But I've come to realize that the importance of stepping up to offer an expression of comfort to someone you truly care about should outweigh that selfish fear.

"Please know that I hold you in my thoughts always with gentle and affectionate regard. I hope you and your family will continue to draw strength and comfort from the memories and meaning of the life you and Harvey built together—and that your future will be surrounded by the ongoing experience of God's grace."

Chapter 18

The Goodbyes Continue

Getting through the day is like walking through a mine field of... moments of recollection. Just when I have slipped beneath the surface of remembering, drawn by the benevolent distractions of daily life, the grim new reality suddenly explodes around me, reminding me that everything is terribly, permanently different. And I must absorb the same first brutal shock, the same descending horror, over and over again. I am deceived by those instances of forgetfulness, yet I am obviously not ready to live every moment with the inalterable truth.

Molly Fumia, *Safe Passage: Words to Help the Grieving*

Dreams, Tributes, and Kayaks

One night about a week after the funeral, I visited the skilled nursing unit in which Harvey had died. When the nurse who had been in charge the night of his death saw me coming down the hall, she called out my name and rushed to hug me. "I'm so glad you came! I really wanted to see you again." We sat down, and I was able to ask her the questions I couldn't ask on that other night as he lay still in the bed. She wept as she explained what happened during those hours, how many times he pressed the call button and how many times he thanked them for responding, how he wanted to get out of bed, how cold he felt, how he called for me. How good the other nurses had been. How the medics pulled him to the floor, unwrapped his blankets and tried to keep his heart going, but it kept stopping again. "I wish I had called you, but we didn't think he would die! I went to the church the next day," she said, "and I prayed about it. I'm so sorry. I didn't know he was going to die!" I was able to comfort and reassure her that she did the best she could and to thank her for her good care and her kindness

In the weeks following Harvey's death, both Ann and our seven-year-old granddaughter experienced strongly symbolic dreams. Our granddaughter dreamed that she was sitting in a shopping cart in Sunday school as the other children were attaching paper butterflies to the wall. But she went out into a hallway to pick out a book. One book had a cover with her name on it. When she turned to the inside, she discovered a message to her from Granddaddy that read, "I love you." She couldn't understand the rest of the inscription, but she knew he was saying that he would always be with her.

Soon after that, Ann dreamed that the family was having lunch at an outdoor café, laughing, talking, and joking, as always. Her dad stood up and said he was going for a walk. She told him that she wanted to come, too, but she had left her shoes at Adam's house (her future husband) and would run and get

The Goodbyes Continue

them. Her dad started out for his walk and, when Ann returned, he was out of sight.

I did not have those dreams. I felt wooden and out of sync. For me, accepting Harvey's death has been like trying to look at the sun: you turn your eyes toward it, but you just can't quite go there—the glare is unbearable. Even so, my fear has been that, if I ever stop grieving, I will lose him completely. I wasn't sure I wanted to "move on," and I certainly did not want to be told that I needed to do so. Grief connects us with the person we have loved, and we can't give it up.

Over time, the cards, food, and dinner invitations came to an end. I participated in a couple of small grief groups and tried to resume my regular activities, including physical therapy for my shoulder, for which I would undergo another surgery in the months ahead. I arranged lunches with married friends and dinners with single friends. I resumed a couple of volunteer activities. I also had business to take care of. I sorted through papers and worked through estate matters. We could have made this task easier had we kept all our records in one place and communicated more effectively. I guess we always thought we would have more time. I had to weed through boxes of files—well-kept, thank goodness—from his office as well as records in our home files. But with the help of trusted advisors, I soon filed the estate documents.

Then Easter came, and Harvey's birthday, and the sadness I felt was more profound than ever. And I know the children felt the same way. Though we continued to laugh over memories of old Dad, it was still hard to believe we would never see him again.

Easter, 2016
Ann's Facebook Post

Many times these Facebook memories appear and show posts I made or pictures I posted of my dad. I am glad I made those posts. But significantly more times than not, my heart drops out of my chest at the sight of them. Last year was my last Easter getting to hold my dad's hand in church. It is hard to remember that the amount of the love in my life has not changed, even though my dad, self-proclaimed president of the Ann Cosper Fan Club, is no longer here. Life is much harder on this April fifth than it was on the last, and I am glad I did not know last year how this feels. But God and I are working on it.

June 8, 2016
Ann's Facebook Post

June is tough this year. My dad's birthday is the thirteenth, and of course, there's my first Father's Day without the first man I ever loved. It is only appropriate that the Mecklenburg County Courthouse is holding court on the thirtieth at 1 p.m. for a memorial for my dad, and I invite anyone so inclined to attend. I will be one of the speakers.

After that, we will be scattering his ashes in Masonboro Sound, where he often took his small fishing boat to troll for bluefish and Spanish mackerel. When discussing where he wanted his ashes, he said that this would be the only way he would catch any fish. #dadquote

The Goodbyes Continue

I still can't believe he's gone. There are times I forget and reach for my phone to call him, like this morning. I spent the day in mediation with two other attorneys who worked with my dad and knew him well, and it was wonderful to see their faces light up when I told a funny story about him. I hope through my posts and my #dadquotes and photos, etc., that I help my dad live on. The world deserves to remember him.

In July, six months after the funeral, a judge presided over a special session at the Mecklenburg County Courthouse so that the county bar association could honor Harvey. Close friends, judges, associates, and family members gathered in a courtroom where Harvey had examined jurors, questioned witnesses, delivered closing arguments, and shaken hands with opposing counsel, plaintiffs, and defendants. Several attorneys spoke eloquently, including our daughter and my sister. His closest long-time law partner entered into the permanent record a tribute full of stories, humorous anecdotes, professional accolades, and memories, including these comments: *"In fifteen years of working together, I never once heard Harvey raise his voice or say an unkind word to a co-worker, to a client, to opposing counsel, to anyone…He taught me, and others he mentored over the years, not only how to practice law well, but how to be a good and decent human being while doing so."*

My sister ended her tribute this way: *"Harvey, we know that you are with that other Fisherman, floating on the water with your rod and reel in your hands. Thank you for teaching your followers*

The Defense Rests

how to bait our hooks, cast our lines, and share our fish with others.
   "*The Defense Rests.*"

The following day, our three children and I drove to the coast to carry out Harvey's wishes: he wanted his ashes sprinkled in Masonboro Sound. On high tide, we paddled brightly colored kayaks to the island and stood together in a circle, our arms around each other's shoulders, in a prayer of thanksgiving for this beloved man. Then we poured the white ashes on the ocean, the beach, and the sound, silently watching as they drifted on the breeze into the sand and water.

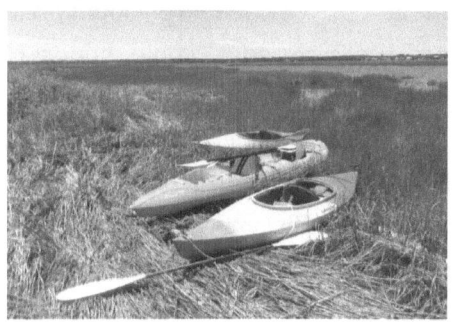

July 9, 2016

SOME CLOTHES ARE STILL IN THE CLOSET

For me, one of the hardest tasks was sorting through Harvey's clothing and possessions. I know some bereaved people who tackled the job right away and others who took years to do it. I have worked in fits and starts, during moments that I felt strong enough, occasionally angry, occasionally weeping, sometimes

The Goodbyes Continue

taking my time and sometimes rushing to get through. After inviting several tall male family members and friends to shop among Harvey's shoes and clothes, I boxed and stacked many items for donation, but much of it remained in the house. I couldn't seem to throw away even a sticky-note with his handwriting on it. I still have his wallet exactly as he left it, including a ten-dollar-bill nestled in the fold.

Once again, like the man at the rest stop on the highway and the man at the appliance store, it was a kind stranger who helped and comforted me when I needed it. One hot day about seven months after Harvey died, I suddenly went on a tear around the house. I opened the back of my SUV and began throwing in shirts, suits, and slacks still on the hangers. I grabbed boxes of shoes and caps and belts and socks and threw them into the back of the car. Then, I drove to a charity thrift shop, by myself, crying the whole way.

An older man was assisting a customer at the front desk when I burst in, wiping my cheeks with the back of my hand and asking where to bring in donations. He calmly directed me to the loading zone around back. I felt sorry for the young woman who came out to help me unload; as I continued to weep, she just didn't know what to say. How could she understand about the Saturday evenings my husband had spent grilling out in the driveway while wearing the red striped polo shirt? How could she imagine the communion bread tasted while he was wearing the gray flannel pants, or the ocean salt water spraying the blue and white bathing suit, or the socks that stretched over those long feet propped on the green plaid ottoman after a long day?

But the older man—he understood. As he slipped around back to help hang the suits, he smiled at me and said, "Forty-six extra-long, right?" I looked at him in surprise: "How did you know?" I asked. "I've been doing this a long time," he said. Then he hugged me and told me that God was with me and I would be okay. After I started the engine of my empty car to depart, he was not surprised when I threw open the door and ran back for the red striped shirt. He probably knew that I would hold it to my face all the way home.

Even today, several years later, I still have some of Harvey's clothes—and that's okay. I can decide about those when I am ready to. As our daughter planned her wedding without her beloved Dad to give her away, a friend turned his soft white fishing shirt into a ring bearer's pillow for a little grandson to carry, while one of his ties wound its way into her bouquet—just two of the ways we honored his presence with us.

Bursts of Grief and Water

Death, like illness, does not happen in a vacuum. There is so much to do after a family member dies that we can't just sit around, bereft, as much as we might want to. In addition to a heavy sadness and lingering sense of disbelief that stayed with me day and night, I found that grief can come in bursts that are entirely unpredictable: a song, a sight, a word, an innocent remark, a random memory can evoke a sudden response of tears. An item of Harvey's might stimulate a memory of the

The Goodbyes Continue

time he purchased it or the last time he touched it. The sight of his beautiful handwriting—which he agreed was as illegible as if a chicken had landed on an ink blotter—or his briefcase—as much as I had sometimes resented it—might send me into sobs.

Meanwhile, the everyday responsibilities of home, pets, cars, and bills had to be taken care of. Life moved on, whether or not I wanted it to. And then came another emergency at the coast.

A few months after the funeral, on the evening before Ann and I were leaving on a much-anticipated trip with a group of Carolina alumni, I received a frantic call from my Wilmington neighbors, who were standing in two inches of water in my kitchen. During a routine check of the house, they found that the water heater upstairs had been overflowing for who-knows-how-long, the kitchen ceiling had sagged almost to the floor, and the walls were caving under waterfalls. Late at night, I had to contact my homeowners insurance carrier, then a construction supervisor and friend who had handled the previous problem, who contracted with a disaster company, who sent a truck to load up nearly everything in the house and take it to a storage facility. Once again, as I had been throughout Harvey's illness, I was blessed with a person in my life who helped me through. Having construction management as a second career, he supervised the entire job, cheerfully handling all the details with professionalism, diligence, sensitivity, patience, and caring. He told me to go ahead on the trip while the house dried out and we'd talk when I returned.

This experience reinforced what I had learned when Harvey became so sick: no matter what we are struggling with, life goes on, with all of its complications. We are walking in mismatched shoes. And, when we are fragile emotionally, making decisions is more difficult. Therapists call it responsibility fatigue. I didn't even want to decide what to eat, or where; if I were dining out with a friend, I wanted her just to tell me where to be, and when. It also reinforced that good people tend to make themselves available to help out just when they are needed most.

I spent much of the next six months on the phone and in the car, making scores of decisions as the house in Wilmington was torn up and put back together: selecting cabinets, flooring, carpet, and paint colors; interviewing window installers, placing electrical outlets, designing a pantry, inspecting materials, waiting for people to show up, paying their bills and then submitting the expenses to the insurance company. Remodeling a twenty-three-year-old house might have been fun—sort of—before Harvey died, but now I didn't much care. I just wanted it to be finished. Thankfully, my contractor friend did most of the coordinating. By the time the restoration was completed, I had dipped into savings once again, and the insurance company had paid out more than eighty thousand dollars. And then, of course, my rates went up.

All this time, what I really wanted to do was just sit and be sad.

Part 5

When Life Goes On

You will lose someone you can't live without, and your heart will be badly broken, and the bad news is that you never completely get over the loss of your beloved. But this is also the good news. They live forever in your broken heart that does not seal back up. And you come through. It's like having a broken leg that never heals perfectly—that still hurts when the weather gets cold, but you learn to dance with the limp.

Anne Lamott, *Stitches*

Chapter 19

Living With Grief

The reality is that you will grieve forever. You will not get over the loss of a loved one; you will learn to live with it. You will heal and you will rebuild yourself around the loss you have suffered. You will be whole again but you will never be the same. Nor should you be the same, nor would you want to.

Elisabeth Kubler-Ross

Grief is not a task to finish
And move on,
But an element of yourself –
An alteration of your being.
A new way of seeing.
A new definition of self.

Gwen Flowers, Grief

The Defense Rests

The Many Ways We Grieve

In 1969, Swiss psychologist Elisabeth Kubler-Ross published a book, *On Death and Dying*, in which she detailed five stages of grief that, according to her research, patients went through when they were diagnosed with a terminal illness. The stages, which she increased to seven in a later work called *On Grief and Grieving*, were eventually shown to be common emotional reactions following the death of someone we love, as well: shock, denial, anger, bargaining, depression, testing, and acceptance. It's helpful to recognize that these aspects of grief are normal. Unfortunately, some people mistakenly interpreted the book to mean that grief was a definitive process of steps to be taken in a certain order to "get through it" and "move on."

The truth is that grief is not an orderly process—not something we eventually pass through and "get over." Grief is complex, messy, life-changing, and life-long. For people who are grieving, life can get easier over time, but time does not magically heal, and there is no set prescription for healing. We do not "move on" from it, but we can move forward, over time. Grief becomes part of us as we learn to move around in a different life.

There are scores of common responses to the death of a loved one, from anxiety to avoidance, disorganization to dread, guilt to hopelessness, loneliness to rage. Many people experience physical symptoms such as shortness of breath and insomnia. We might feel as if we are going crazy. We wonder how we are to continue living. We might want to go to bed with the covers over our heads. But, unless we become so depressed that we cannot function in everyday life, or feel suicidal—in which case we must seek immediate help—we find our own individual keys to mourning, grieving, and some kind of acceptance, over time.

For example, an extrovert is more likely to seek company, whereas an introvert needs more time alone. We might be afraid that our emotional responses, our frequent tears, will make other people uncomfortable. Or we might be afraid others will judge us if we are not crying—trying to get on with normal activities. In the months and years following the loss of someone we love, most of us find that—like a ringing in the ears—the pain does not go away, but we grow more accustomed to it.

Ask any widow or widower about loneliness and, chances are, you will see tears. When we lose the person with whom we have shared our lives, we are missing a part of ourselves. We feel a heavy, profound sadness that only people who have had such a loss can understand. I was afraid that nothing would ever take away the loneliness that seemed only to grow deeper. It was different from the difficult loss of my mother and father in the previous decade. I can only imagine the loss of a child or a sibling. Even while the stages of grief might be definable, the experience is unique for each of us.

Every day, more than once, when I think about losing Harvey, my breath catches and my body freezes and I want to believe he's not really gone from this physical, earthly life.

SUGGESTIONS FOR THOSE GRIEVING THE LOSS OF A LOVED ONE

- One key to surviving the death of someone we love is to **give ourselves permission to mourn and grieve in our own ways.** It shocks us over and over again that the person we loved is really gone, that there is nothing anyone can do to change it or make it better. I had to **acknowledge that no one else is ever going to fix it,** and I would have to accept my own feelings and find my own way to survive without him. We have to somehow reach a level of acceptance, no matter what form or how long it takes. And that means we need to be gentle and patient with ourselves.
- **Importantly, we must take care of our physical selves.** Especially after a long illness in which we have been exhausted caregivers, we can plan physical activities and maintain eating habits that improve our health: schedule workouts several times a week, invite a friend to join us for regular walks, or fill the refrigerator with fresh fruits and vegetables.
- **We can find ways to relax and be comforted.** I spent some time at the beach, writing, reading, sleeping late, planting flowers, swimming, browsing consignment shops, and—when I needed company—visiting with friends. I walked to the Intracoastal Waterway, where I could watch the tiny crabs scuttling in and out with the tide and the pelicans diving for fish; I could hear the gulls arguing over which one owned the top of a post leading to the marina; and I could smell the salty spray as boats sped

by. I wept as I thought of Harvey out there in his boat, before, and his ashes out there where he wanted them to be, now—part of God's ageless creation.

- **Pet companions—the ones we already have or, when we feel ready, new ones—can provide us with comfort, amusement, love, and fun.** I have been comforted by the companionship of my dogs, who walk with me every day, follow me around the house, sit with me on the back porch, and sleep in my bedroom—or bed.
- As a Christian, I find solace in **praying, both alone and with other people**, though some days it was—and still is —difficult. Throughout my life, and especially in the past few years, I have been comforted by scripture passages, especially reciting over and over the Twenty-third Psalm; I had memorized it as a child with the help of my mother, and it has helped me throughout my life:

"The Lord is my shepherd; I shall not want...Yea, though I walk through the valley of the shadow of death, I will fear no evil, for thou art with me. Thy rod and thy staff, they comfort me...Surely goodness and mercy shall follow me all the days of my life, and I will dwell in the house of the Lord forever."

- **There are many helpful programs, support groups, therapists, counselors, and books on grief.** Some churches offer support through **Stephen Ministry** programs, in which lay leaders are trained to be supportive, listening Christian friends during hard times. I attended short-term group sessions at a retirement center, then an all-day widows' retreat at the church. I participated in a Christian **GriefShare** program for several months. The videos, workbook, discussion, and sharing with new friends who were grieving were very helpful, though the theology undergirding the program was different from mine and that of my denomination.

- Even when we want to talk to no one, or—the opposite—think and talk about nothing else except our grief, there comes a time—there come times in spurts or waves—to **accept and seek out fellowship with others**. Even when we don't feel like it, or feel guilty having any fun at all without the person we have lost. We might choose people who are suffering through similar losses. Or we might choose people and activities unrelated to loss at all. We do well to choose people with whom we can be ourselves, who can cry with us, who can make us laugh. On the first anniversary of Harvey's death, I invited seven widowed friends to my home for dinner. Since most did not know each other, I prepared a corny icebreaking game, a sheet of paper on which they filled in names beside descriptions such as "I retired from many years of working in a bank and am now a fierce competitor at the bridge table," and "I am a voiceover artist who moved to this area last year from New York to be near my daughter." It was months later that I realized I had served the same foods that Harvey had eaten on his last night, exactly one year earlier.

I am also part of a new widows' group forming at church. I invited the grandchildren over on some Friday nights for "Dinner at Deedee's" while their parents enjoyed a date night together.

- **We can go back to work or to volunteer activities we have enjoyed.** In a way, I envied my widowed friends who were still working, because they had a specific reason to get up in the morning and prescribed activities to distract them during the day. Others have found different jobs or part-time work to be fulfilling. I was retired from grant-writing and no longer interested in a career. But my long-time activities including choir, reading to children at a local school, various volunteer commitments, Bible study groups, and regular group lunches with friends have been a solace.
- When we lose our best companions, it's difficult to see other couples together. We experience pangs of longing and envy when others are holding hands as they leave a concert or enjoying a meal at a restaurant together. Like forcing ourselves to jump into the chilly water of a swimming pool, however, **we can decide to spend time around other couples**, grow accustomed to the initial discomfort, and be happy for them. After all, they did not cause our loss. It helps **not to idealize the people and relationships we no longer have**; others surely have disagreements and problems, as we did with our loved ones. We can only hope they realize how fortunate they are to have each other.

- At some point, when we are ready, it's helpful to **make a list of all the things we have always wanted to do, a "bucket list" of activities**—reasonable and affordable, or not—and examine what that list tells us about the ways we can build a future without the person we have lost.
- Among the widows I know, many of us embarked on **home improvement projects**, even small ones, that fit into our budgets. A year after the renovations at the coast were completed, I decided to remodel our outdated master bathroom and had the upstairs of the house repainted for the first time in many years. My widowed friends were embarking on similar projects with an eye toward eventually down-sizing, but also for another reason. As one friend said, "I think subconsciously I was accepting that my husband was really not coming back. I began making the house mine instead of ours. And that was a good thing."
- **We can make some new memories.** Taking a trip with someone we enjoy is a wonderful diversion, even it's a day trip to a fun or beautiful place. My daughter and I have laughed and cried our way through vacation trips with Carolina alumni, and we are still reliving the experiences we had and relishing the new stories we continue to tell.
- **We can process memories and express ourselves creatively through photo books and collections, writing, sewing, and other projects suited to our interests and abilities.**
- **We can make new friends.** Common experiences can

help us to bond. In social interactions, I have more in common now with single women and widows than I have with married couples, and we enjoy dinners, trips, and events together, sometimes one-on-one and sometimes in groups.

- **We can work to make sure that the needs of other grieving people are being met in our communities.** I know of a widow who started a support ministry through her church; it has now grown to include not only social events but other services provided free of charge by volunteers: counseling, home repairs, referrals, financial advice, children's support, and more. Some friends and I are working with church staff and others to start a Surviving Our Spouses (SOS) group for fellowship, programs, and outreach. We recognize that truly meaningful initiatives on behalf of bereaved people include individualized support, because each person's needs are unique.
- **We can continue to find ways to honor the person who has died, keeping the loved one alive in our conversations, our memories, and our hearts.** Our daughter walked down the aisle at her wedding between her two brothers as she held the bouquet wrapped with one of her dad's favorite ties. When the minister asked who gave this woman to be married to this man, I was able to say "Her father and I" as the altar candles glowed in loving memory and gratitude for his life, and we felt his presence among us.

Chapter 20

A Widow Writes to Her Husband

> *What we have once enjoyed we can never lose. All that we love deeply becomes a part of us.*
>
> Helen Keller

As people who are grieving, we must find our own best ways to face and process what we have lost. During those first months, I found comfort in writing to Harvey. Though I never planned on sharing them, I now know that these letters express some thoughts and feelings that are common among bereaved people. Once again, they reflect the world of contradictory realities that we live in: sadness, regret, guilt and despair…along with gratitude, appreciation, comfort…and, over time, even something approaching acceptance.

March 13, 2016 – Communion

Twelve weeks. It's been twelve weeks since I saw you for the last time. I see you in my memory, my imagination, pictures, family videos, but I will never see you here in the flesh again.

The Defense Rests

I wept through Communion today. The kind of weeping others don't notice unless they're looking right at you, unless they know you very well. We take the Lord's Supper with sorrow in confessing our own unworthiness. We take it with gratitude for the grace we have been given by God through Christ. Sometimes I am imagining that first Last Supper and all that was happening in the life of Jesus. Communion is, after all, for us Christians an experience of active remembrance.

But today I wept through Communion in remembrance of you. I looked out from my seat in the choir loft at the pew, empty today, in which you sat for so many years with the children, passing the bread and cup. Where once—an oft-told family story—after the children had taken to the altar the bread we had baked to serve the congregation, you sat on the bread basket and crushed it, causing you all to laugh your way quietly and guiltily through the rest of the service, shoulders shaking. (I heard this from the ladies who sat behind you.) I looked out at the elders' pews, from which you had filed forward so many times to the altar to pick up the trays to serve the congregation. You always looked so nice in your dark suit, and I loved the barely perceptible wink you gave me up there in the choir loft as you slipped past.

I wept through Communion as I remembered the first time the elders came to serve you in the hospital after the stroke. You had the feeding tube, so they gently touched your closed lips with the bread and cup as they read the ancient words of Jesus at the Last Supper. And I wept because I remembered your final Communion, as you lay in the skilled nursing bed, the elders serving us the elements, how strong your voice sounded as we all prayed The Lord's Prayer together. We could not have known it would be your last. I wept in the most profound grief for you, for Jesus, for suffering and death and what it does to us. And I wept in gratitude for what Communion affirmed —for you, for me, for all of us: that death is not the final answer for the life of the soul.

June 13, 2016 – Happy Birthday

Your birthday. The first June thirteenth in sixty-nine years (counting the day you were born) that you have not been alive on this earth. Six days from now, our three children will celebrate Father's Day without their dad for the first time.

It comes near the six-month mark following your death, at a time when I am eating almost all of my meals alone—in fact, when I am almost always alone. When the house phone rings, it is mostly with calls from telemarketers or home repair people working on our wrecked house in Wilmington. When people think I should be getting better day by day, or "moving on" even though I had not gone a single day in forty-five years without the person I loved who knew me the best and loved me anyway.

But it's not mostly about me. It's about you. It's about what you suffered for so many months, how hard the end of your life was, the pain and disappointment and frustration I fear you tried to hide, and how you still believed you were "the most blessed man on the planet" and didn't want it to end, even then. It's about the all the things you are missing. Thinking that "he's in a better place" doesn't help much, because you aren't here, with me, with the people you loved and who loved you, doing the things you wanted to do before you died.

The Defense Rests

I am not without gratitude—huge mountains of gratitude for the blessings of your life and of our life together. I am not without hope—small glimmers of hope that, over time, getting through the day will become easier, and the big black hole will start to close bit-by-bit, and life will take on renewed meaning. You left me with so much to remember and to be thankful for, including family, friends, and resources for a comfortable life. But you left me without you. Wherever you are, Harvey Cosper, on this birthday, I am sorry you died; but, most important, I am glad you lived.

Labor Day 2016 – For a Man at Rest

What would we be doing today, you and I, if you were here? Probably we would be at the beach. You would have gotten up early to fish out in the ocean on the Defense Rests, while I walked the dogs, putzed around the house, read a book on the porch swing. When you returned, with or without a catch, you would have cleaned off your fishing rods and lined them up in the garage along with the other nine or ten. You would have emerged from the shower and put on another pair of khaki shorts, a clean old tee shirt and those brown rubber sandals with the striped laces in an x pattern on the top. Then we would have put some hot dogs on the grill. That would have been many of the forty-five Labor Days we had together. A day of fun and rest, apart from the thousands of days of hard work that you did so well and so cheerfully, on behalf of others. And what about all those Labor Day weekends we spent in the mountains with our college friends, floating down the New River in our big black rubber tubes, drinking lukewarm beer and laughing and talking, then showering at the local gym, eating the favorite dishes we prepared every year, playing golf and tennis, sneaking off to our rooms, then partying late into the night?

Last year on Labor Day, you were lying in a nursing home bed that was too short for you, the sounds of a woman hollering and cursing around the corner. You were covered with an itchy red rash. You couldn't sit up or turn over without assistance. We were waiting anxiously to learn whether a nice retirement community would accept you, since we knew you could never come home again. But we were together.

We could not have imagined then that, before the next Labor Day, the kids and I would be holding your ashes in a clear plastic bag inside a cardboard box inside a red velvet bag, nestled in a kayak as we crossed the waterway to our favorite little island. That we, the four people who loved you most in the world, would pray together over the bags and the box, then empty them as the sand, the wind, and the water took you to themselves. I believe you were there, watching us and loving us.

So now it's Labor Day again. We still have your briefcase, the one that took so many files into courtrooms. The one that Hank marked when you set it down after work. There are still some shirts and ties in the closet and boat cushions in the garage. At once feeling your enormous presence and your enormous absence, I sit alone at a table for six and look out into the yard where you broke your thumb playing baseball with the kids. Where you strung up a rope between trees to teach your daughter to bat. Where you mowed the grass and planted shrubs and your dad taught the boys to "water" the bushes when you guys thought no one else was looking. There is a nip of fall in the breeze, bright sunshine, leaves trembling, and the whirring of cicadas, swelling and ebbing. I have nothing to do, no place to go, no reason to open the grill, even if I knew how to use it. I think of all those afternoons, those years, when a Labor Day—a day free from work—was a gift. Now I would give almost anything to be in your car on the way to the hardware store, or washing your stained and hole-y Rock and Roll Hall of Fame tee shirt, rinsing mustard off the blue and white dishes, or even reading aloud at your bedside while aides change the dressings on your tattered arms.

"For all the saints, who from their labors rest," we sang at your memorial service. This year Labor Day has a whole new meaning, one I had never thought of before. It marks the ultimate rest for your good labor and, we trust, the ultimate peace that has come to a faithful man after a life well-lived.

November 2016 – All-Saints Day

Today your name was read from a list of church members who have died in the past year. After each name, the organ chimed one bell. Since I couldn't manage to sing the poignant words of the requiem with the choir, I sat out in the congregation. After the names were read, we filed forward for Holy Communion to dip the cubes of bread into the chalice of grape juice. Then we placed the spiky white flowers into vases in memory of our loved ones. In numbness and sorrow, I placed my flower for you, as did many of our friends.

Before the service, I ran into an older friend with memory

problems who had attended your funeral last year. He said, "How's Harvey?" I stopped cold and stared at him. After a few seconds, I responded, "Harvey's fine. He's doing fine."

As I walked ahead, I realized that it was true: you are fine. Of course you are. It's me who isn't fine. You left me with so much. The memory of your voice, your touch, your hands, your laugh, your face. A thousand treasures to last more than a lifetime. But you left me. And, oh God, what I miss is just you.

January 13, 2017 – Double Anniversary

So we made it through December nineteenth, the first anniversary of your death, and what would have been our forty-sixth wedding anniversary. In spite of several invitations from the children and from friends, I elected to stay home alone. I listened to the classical music you loved and baked my usual Christmas cinnamon bread. At midday, Graham texted with an offer to bring lunch. He arrived with an armload of the traditional red flowers with a little card quoting the floral delivery guy: "Have a GREAT day!" We sat at the table together, he in your regular seat, eating subs and chips and reminiscing about you. I think he needed to do this as much as I did. In the evening, when I couldn't accept their supper invitation because my bread was still in the works, he and the kids stopped by with hot Krispy Kreme doughnuts.

When memories are both so good and so bad, you're on a roller coaster of emotions. I remembered our Carolina days of dating at the DU house, dancing, laughing with friends, driving those ridiculous old Corvairs, buying the cheapest beer at the drive-through, *and watching Dr. Paul Bearer introduce funny horror movies. I remembered the day of our wedding, a short and tame affair with lunch afterwards at the church. Who can truly fathom forty-five years as partners, the growing family, the loving and the disagreeing, the long-running inside jokes, the movies and songs we could quote by heart, the family dramas, church services, multiple cars, four different houses we lived in, pets from dogs to hermit crabs to guinea pigs, trips to the beach and across the sea, the ceremonies, the thousands of meals, the choices and decisions, prayers, ball games, school plays and concerts, the things we said and the things we didn't say, and the work—always your work. And, toward the end, your illness and pain, the hospital rooms, the falls, the bloody walls, the wheelchairs, somehow still looming larger right now than most of the other forty-plus years of better health.*

The hardest moment of this one-year anniversary was leaving our beautiful Christmas Service of Lessons and Carols and realizing, as I walked through the parking lot at sunset, that I had lived one year to the exact moment from the last time that I saw you alive. You had eaten supper. You were propped up in bed talking about buying a truck. Never mind that you couldn't drive, or walk, or stand, or even sit up by yourself. You always had hope.

I had placed my hands on the back of your neck and on your cheek as I kissed you goodbye, ever the busy one making sure you had everything you needed—call button, drink, cell phone, TV remote, book—within your reach. "Love you," we said. I paused at the door: "See you in the morning."

A Widow Writes to Her Husband

April 4, 2017 – It's Raining

Rain is falling on the pink cherry blossoms beyond our covered porch out back. The petals are feathering onto the weathered cover of your car, which is still parked in the driveway next to mine. Your nemesis Hank, the very old "devil dog" you loved to hate, is snoring inside a blanket beside me. Clothes are clicking in the dryer and the house smells like spaghetti sauce with sausage, the way you always liked it.

The problem is that you aren't here. And you won't be coming home. Not after work, not for dinner. Not ever again. The void looms; it's too big to take in. And sometimes, like spring storms tearing down the flowers, I can't stop the regrets from coming.

Next week will be the fourth anniversary of the stroke. So it's been four years since I heard you come in the back door after a long day at work. Since you kissed me hello as I held your cheeks in my palms, and then you went upstairs to change out of your suit into jeans. Since I poured you a glass of wine as you propped sideways on a stool at the kitchen counter while I was cooking supper and asked, "So what went on today?" And yet, I still wait for you. I still listen for your car.

It's been almost two years since you lived in this house and sixteen months since you died. Most of your clothes have gone to thrift shops and to friends larger than your children. Your Bible, your gold cross, your watches and your law books are with the kids. But your wallet is just as you left it. Your hairbrush still sits in the bathroom drawer, where I can take it out to hold and hang on to your scent. Your favorite books and CDs are right where you left them. Your old tackle box and the moldy orange life jackets still sit on the shelf in the garage at the beach, right where you left them. Your retirement income from so many years of hard work is seeping month by month into my checking account to keep me comfortable here—if comfortable is a word that can be used by widows.

I don't know exactly where you are or what you're like now. You aren't appearing to me in dreams. I wish I knew what it's like for you. As a Christian, I am comforted that you are without pain and with the God and the people you have loved.

As for me, can you see me here? Going to Bible study and exercise, getting together with friends, singing in the choir, playing with the grandchildren, emailing jokes with the kids, all of us laughing at the funny things you said? Do you see me trying to have fun even though you are gone? Having friends over for a birthday lunch and being the odd number at the table, saying the blessing in your place? Do you see me eating alone at a TV tray night after night? Are emanations of love and grief wafting up to you?

I miss you more than I ever thought possible. The shock of realization can physically take away my breath, again and again, every day. But, as you always predicted, I really am getting along okay. Extroverts tend to seek out others, and that helps a lot. You and I have been blessed with many good friends. Most days hold plenty of people and activities and even some laughter. If only I could control the regret.

For instance, I regret that I didn't always fix our deviled eggs with pickles, the way you liked them—and regret even more than I made fun of you about liking them that way. I regret that you found your clean undershirts back in the dresser drawer folded inside-out for thirty years, in protest, because I couldn't convince

A Widow Writes to Her Husband

you to put them in the laundry basket right-side-out. I regret that I was practical and busy instead of gentle and relaxed. I regret that I complained about the neon blue Corvette you were so proud of, even though you could barely fold your big body into it. Why didn't I just enjoy it with you and ask for rides with the top down? I regret so many little things that I said and did, neglected to say and do, over the years. I can only pray that my caregiving in those last hard months showed, more than anything, the depth of my love.

I regret that you suffered so much. Disability, pain, being poked and prodded and moved around until you wanted to cry out to be left alone, and, especially, the indignity of it all. It was so hard to see. It still is.

And I regret this so very much: I didn't follow your lead to talk to you about your death. About a month before you died, you told me that you didn't think you would live much longer, and I didn't encourage you to tell me about that. In my typical optimistic avoidance, I told you that you didn't have anything life-threatening right then, and I dismissed what you were telling me. Why, why did I not respond, "So what are you thinking? How does that feel?" and free you to talk about it?

Why did I not seize the opportunity to talk about what dying might mean to each of us, being apart, what you expected and hoped for when that happened? Because the night that you died, the nurse told me you had been talking to me for hours. She said it sounded as though you were "giving instructions" to Kandy. "We didn't expect him to die," she exclaimed through tears, "or we would have called you sooner." By the time they called me to come, it was too late. What were your instructions? What did you want me to know? I am afraid this not knowing will plague me for the rest of my life.

The greatest regret of all, of course, is not for me but for you—you and the children, who miss you more than you could imagine, and the grandchildren, who are no longer making new memories with you. You missed out on working until you were ready to leave, the easy days of retirement, growing old together, adding to your tome of funny sayings we continue to quote and enjoy, seeing your children settled into secure middle age, growing a garden, learning to play the piano and improving at guitar, cooking new dishes, listening to music, tinkering with an old car or boat, taking trips, sleeping late, and finishing your memoirs—all the things you planned on doing. Cheering on the grandchildren at their concerts and sporting events and helping the youngest to catch his first fish. Visiting all the major league baseball parks. Mentoring Ann as she follows in your footsteps in the law and walking her down the aisle at her wedding. Visiting David's university classes and sharing your mutual love of music, books, movies, and teaching. Going to Kenya to "help" Graham as he trains pediatric surgeons. Watching the Panthers play in the Super Bowl and the Tar Heels win the national championship again—the Heels won! Did you know that? I cheered alone in our bonus room surrounded by our Carolina memorabilia, where we had screamed through so many games together. All of this would be richer, fuller, more fun, if you were here with us. You would have just loved it, all of it.

The deep hole you left will never be filled. I pray that God will help me deal with these regrets and bring peace, as I pray he has brought peace to you. You enriched us, and you enrich us still. Your love lives on.

Chapter 21

The Time After

I believe that God wants us to know deeply in our souls that we are not alone, that there is a reality bigger than our reality, and that, in that reality, we will find the meaning and purpose of our lives.

Dr. Robert W. Henderson,
"*Send Me?*" sermon, Covenant Presbyterian Church,
January 13, 2019

Responding to Grieving Friends in the Months and Years after a Death

If there's anything I would tell you, as someone who's walked through the Grief Valley, it is that the time your presence is most needed and most powerful is in those days and weeks and months and years after the funeral; when most people have withdrawn and the road is most isolating. It is in the countless ordinary moments that follow, when grief suckerpunches you and you again feel it all fully.

The Defense Rests

> *...Remind yourself to reach out to people long after the services and memorials have concluded.*
> *Death is a date on the calendar, but grief is the calendar.*
>
> John Pavlovitz,
> https://johnpavlovitz.com, the-grieving-you-need-most-after-the-funeral, January 5, 2005, blog

When we lose someone we love, we appreciate those friends who **allow us to grieve in our own way, in our own time.** People who **don't expect us to "get over it" or "move on,"** because we will grieve for the rest of our lives. Even as our feelings of loss become less intense, less all-consuming, they do not go away. We appreciate those who recognize that mourning is exhausting. I will never forget overhearing some of my parents' friends complaining that a member of their group did not come downstairs to see them when they visited after her daughter died; to this day, this brings tears to my eyes.

It's helpful when people **continue to remember and acknowledge us.** Over time, the mailbox that once was filled with loving cards contains mostly bills and solicitations. **Phone calls and messages to "see how you're getting along"** dwindle, then stop. People see you around town and assume you're getting along just fine. For me, in those first months, I missed my husband with a physical pain, and I was living alone for the first time in my life. The enormity of the loss and change was difficult to fathom. The sadness consumed me, and I was not very good company. I felt impatient. Subjects that had previously made for interesting conversation seemed mundane and silly; I couldn't talk about the news, because I wasn't keeping up. It was hard to concentrate on reading or television. Music made me sad. But I found that I needed friends just as much, if not more, after the funeral. I learned that it means a great deal when people continue to remember. We appreciate **being encouraged to accept invitations but not being pressured** if we don't feel like going out at the time.

In a recent survey of surviving spouses, I asked: "What is the most helpful, comforting thing that others said or did for you when you lost your spouse?" The responses I received varied, of course, but one overriding theme was this: **grieving people want to hear about the person they lost**. Hearing the loved one's name is important. **Occasional cards and notes, even comments in passing** at the grocery store, bring tears and smiles of comfort. Expressions of love and appreciation, the sharing of memories, stories of how much the person meant to others: these are the greatest gifts of all. Recently, having learned from my own experience, I sought out two mothers whose daughters had gone to Sunday school with my children many years ago. One had died as a preschooler and one as a teenager. I shared with each mother what I fondly remembered about her girl. Each cried tears of gratitude. Each said no one had mentioned her child in many years.

Holidays and special occasions are difficult following the death of a loved one. The next Christmas is not merry and the next birthday is not happy. For me, even though I look forward to receiving Christmas pictures of joyful intact families having fun together, those cards also make me sad. For the first two

Christmases after Harvey died, I sent cards with current, smiling family pictures on the front and a picture of Harvey on the back, above a quote from the Bible. I have been especially grateful for friends who **acknowledge the difficulty of special occasions**: "I know this day is a hard one for you." Or, "This time of year must be especially difficult for you. We will always remember Harvey." Two of Harvey's sisters continue to send me cards for Valentine's Day and other special occasions. Just knowing that someone else sympathizes is comforting when you no longer have a valentine sweetheart with whom to celebrate—even if he usually just stopped at the drugstore on the way home for a box of candy on sale and a funny card while you cooked his favorite foods for a late dinner.

As the months of loneliness stretch on, we appreciate those who **invite us to come over or to go out** but who understand if we need to stay home on especially hard days. And we appreciate people who say, **"I am going to call you to get together" and actually follow through on the promise as soon as possible.**

My survey of grieving friends reinforced this universal truth: as time goes on, fewer and fewer invitations come our way. Friends often feel awkward inviting a single person to a group filled with couples, for example. And it's true that, as the fifth wheel, the single person can feel awkward, too. But fun and conversation can help overcome any unease people might feel. **It's best to be open and honest about how to handle invitations and social situations.** A friend recently asked me whether, when she invites a recently widower for dinner with several married couples, she should include another single person. I knew how I would feel if I were the odd man out (please don't), but I told her, "Just ask him what would be most comfortable for him."

Finally, it's normal for grieving people to find themselves less focused, and more distracted or forgetful, than usual—especially those of us who had those tendencies to begin with, augmented by the effects of growing older. We appreciate **patience and humor** as we try to get our act together and keep it together.

> September 16, 2016
> Kandy's Facebook Post
> Subject: Going crazy is normal
>
> First I lost my Kindle. It was not in the car or the doctor's office. After a month, I ordered a new one. Thankfully, I had just received my replacement Visa card in the mail, prior to finding my old one under the passenger seat in my car days later while looking for my Kindle. Then I lost my favorite pair of shoes, which I found outside in the bushes, underneath a window I had climbed onto a chair to clean. Since they were shrunken and muddy from the rain, and now two different colors, I had to throw them away. I went to the mall to look for a new pair, ate lunch, shopped a bit and, on the way home, had to turn around to go back and look for my cell phone. After a fruitless search through a garbage bin at the food court, I found the phone at a shop where I had left it in a dressing room. Then I realized I didn't have my forty dollars in change from the grocery store checkout the day before. I went back to the store and they confirmed the checker came out forty dollars ahead, so they gave me two twenties. Then

The Defense Rests

this morning the ladies at the manicure place next door to Curves saw me working out and knocked on the window while holding up my long-lost Kindle. I am now heading back to Walmart to get the jug of Tide that I left in the bottom of my cart. Last night I was so relieved at my first GriefShare session to learn that "feeling as if you have lost your mind" is one of the most prominent effects of grief. Although there are some close to me who would argue that none of this is unusual for me. It's been several years since I found a spoon in my glasses case.

A Summary of Lessons Learned

The most beautiful people we have known are those who have known defeat, known suffering, known struggle, known loss, and have found their way out of the depths. These persons have an appreciation, a sensitivity, an understanding of life that fills them with compassion, gentleness, and a deep loving concern. Beautiful people do not just happen.

Elisabeth Kubler-Ross,
AZQuotes.com, Wind and FLY LTD, 2019.
http://www.azquotes.com/quote/395280,
accessed October 8, 2019

The Time After

> *The practice of gratitude confronts our downward spiral tendencies and transforms us into people of radiant possibility, people who used to see disappointment and failure who now see a future filled with hope and new life.*
>
> Dr. Robert W. Henderson,
> *"In All Circumstances?"* sermon series:
> *"With Grateful Hearts,"* Covenant Presbyterian Church,
> March 3, 2019

As I tell our story, I find that I have learned many lessons that would have been valuable to know beforehand. I hope that others will find them valuable, as well. Here are a few that stand out to me.

- If you are a medical or hospital patient, appoint an advocate, work to understand your issues and treatment, and be kind to your caregivers. You always have the opportunity to make a positive difference in the lives of others, even if you are living your life mostly in one room.
- Keep a gratitude journal, on paper, in your head, or in your prayers.
- Exercise, eat well, and get some sleep.
- Keep a current will, living will, and powers of attorney.
- Organize important papers and household records.
- Say "I love you" every day.
- Memorize the Twenty-third Psalm.
- Read out loud.
- Listen to music.
- Beware of old water heaters upstairs.

- When a person you care about shares a deep worry or concern, instead of jumping in with a story about yourself, with words that minimize or deflect, say, "Tell me more about that." Then listen. Even if they want to talk about dying.
- Pray together.
- Laugh. A lot. Find the humor in situations and don't take yourself too seriously.
- Allow yourself to take one day at a time.
- Encourage the sharing of memories (What was your favorite car? Remember that trip we made?).
- Listen patiently to the flywheel stories. One day you will miss them and the person who tells them.
- Choose positive people and ask them to call or visit or have dinner.
- Keep your mind sharp through conversation, puzzles, books, outings, and games.
- Say all the things you might not get to say again.
- Hang onto the striped polo shirt as long as you want to.
- Don't criticize or complain about the little things that annoy you. A time might come when you would give anything to make deviled eggs with pickles, just to watch a person you love enjoy eating them.
- Take a deep breath before panicking when something bad happens.
- Tell your story, when you know it's safe—when you are with people who will pay attention and who will honor and protect your story, and you.

The Time After

- Cultivate and display a sense of gratitude for life. It requires discipline and courage to thank God for being there with us no matter what is happening. Thank God for all of life.
- Respond in some way—your own way—to people going through hard times. Find your own way to show compassion. See it as a call. Don't wait for the perfect time. Just do it.
- At no time will any of our lives be all bad or all good; at no time will we be fully prepared for everything that happens. Sometimes our shoes won't match, but that's okay: we have another pair just like them at home.

Deciding to Live Every New Day

Rebelliously, I put out the light in my house,
And Your sky surprised me with its stars.
Rabindranath Tagore, *The Heart of God*

Looking back, I see that we could count on God to send just the right people, just when we needed them. God met us in the people who cared for us—in messages, letters, hugs, and quiet deeds. In the hardest of times, we merely had to wait, because the gifts always came. It could be the friend who stands at the door of the hospital room and smiles. The young man who prays silently at the foot of the bed. The football fan who kneels in front of your chair on the beach. The therapist who slips into an office between appointments to make a difficult telephone call.

The Defense Rests

The bathroom attendant who brings you clean cloths and gentle help without being asked. The minister who calls when you are starting to lose hope to remind you of what is truly important. The appliance salesman mourning for his son who hugs you with tears in his eyes. The man at the thrift shop who hangs up the familiar shirts and holds you as you cry. The neighbor who asks for your toilet brush and the one who drives you to a doctor's office to check on your broken collarbone. The rows of friends behind you in the pews and lining up in the cold just to let you know they are with you. The homemade soup in the freezer and cinnamon bread on the countertop. The hundreds of get-well cards overflowing a basket in the corner.

God is with me in the dark, on my side of the bed at night when the other side is empty, and when I run across Harvey's handwriting on an old card or rummage through his tool box. When my breath catches at the sight of his favorite rocker on the porch and the little orange-painted shop where he ate his last ice cream cone.

So much of life is still hard. I had never lived alone, and it's something I have to get used to. Harvey would not be at all surprised to know that I've started talking to myself—I can just hear him commenting that I never cared before whether anyone else was listening or not.

I am grieving not just for myself, for my best supporter, my accountability, defender, closest friend, and filter on the world. I am grieving for what he lost out on, what our children and grandchildren have lost out on with his not being here. On our third Easter without Harvey, our little grandson, who remembers his grandfather only through stories and pictures, found me in the kitchen and stretched his arms around my waist. "I wish Granddaddy could be here," he said.

I think about the person I was when we were younger, before anyone close to me had died. I felt so cheerful, so lighthearted much of the time. Conversations were full of jokes and affectionate teasing. Then my mother died, and other people I loved. As I grew older, I saw more suffering. Life seemed sadder. Finally, with the death of my husband, I became convinced that I will never again be that carefree person. Always at the back of my mind, and always in my heart, is sorrow too deep to ignore, too deep for words.

When we experience such loss, we become different. We are more self-preserving, more careful to protect ourselves from potentially hurtful people and from situations that can make us especially sad. We are harder in some ways but softer in others. We are better listeners. Tears come more easily. We can see more deeply into a suffering person's soul. Knowing what we now know about suffering, we find within ourselves new wells of sympathy and compassion for ourselves and for others.

It's not just a saying on a tee shirt: life is good. Each season of the year has its unique beauty, from one year to the next. I love, and am loved by, children, grandchildren, family, and friends. I continue many of the ordinary activities I enjoyed before. I play the piano Harvey presented to me as an anniversary surprise not long before the stroke, in a characteristically rare but extravagant burst of generosity, and I remember my last error-filled but heartfelt concert for him— Beethoven, Schumann, Debussy— as he listened from his armchair, head back and eyes closed. I learn to take care of things I didn't know about before—like changing furnace filters, organizing taxes, and hiring roofers. I try to stay busy and grounded.

But I am lonely, and lonely for my husband, and time and busyness will never fill the void. I have to make sure that this is not a double death—because one of us still has some life to live out on this earth. So I have to make the decision every day to get up and move, while permitting myself moments, or days, just to be sad.

This is what I know: we can be bitter or we can be grateful. And I could not be more grateful for the gift of my husband, the life we had together, the life I still have, in large part thanks to him, and the people who have surrounded us with love. The decision to be grateful, as Harvey was, as God bids me to be, is one I that I must make every new day, one day at a time. Already I see, like the moon coming up over Masonboro Island, little shards of joy starting to shimmer through.

"So very sad for you," a friend wrote to me on the day my Harvey died. "Harvey's struggle has been difficult, but the story was love of family and friends and a deep and abiding faith in God. You will continue, and hopefully we will still read your story."

Acknowledgments

My mother, Barbara Murray Perrin, taught me to love words. For years when I was a child, she assigned me a "word of the day" to be spelled and used in sentences: thus, I could be overheard telling my father he was "irascible" and describing myself as "perspicacious" while our "hirsute" dog spent time "reconnoitering" in the yard. Since she left college after two years to marry my dad and gave birth to me thirteen months later, and her own early writing burned up in a house fire, my mom counted on me to become the champion speller and the writer in the family. Reading was a lifetime joy for her. Until not long before she died, she asked me repeatedly, "When are you going to write your book?" Okay, Mom: here it is. I finally found my story to tell.

My father, James R. Perrin, tried without success to get my first writings published when I was very young: "Poems and Stories from the Heart of a Child." He was so proud of his family, and he was a real character; in fact, he might just be the subject of my next book.

I am grateful to my children for more than I can put into words. They were active, pleasant, fun children to raise and became loving, interesting, productive adults. For Harvey and for me, they also became our truest friends. Thanks to Graham, in his direct surgeon's words, and David, in his philosophical professor's words, for telling me that the first draft wasn't the real story from their real mom, and for redirecting me to make it the whole truth and nothing but the truth, told with greater warmth and self-understanding. With ever-present grace, humor, and respect, they found their own best ways to love and support us even as the struggle must have been so hard on them, as well. And thanks to Ann, who could not possibly have supported us any better or loved us any more; her sparkling personality, deep sensitivity, dry wit, and sacrificial loyalty fed our souls, and her contributions to this story are immeasurable.

Thanks to my sister, Jan Perrin Paul, for her constant love, support, encouragement, and humor throughout bad times and good. She was the consummate reader who spent an emotionally exhausting weekend laughing, crying, and editing her heart out until she finally commented, "Okay. You killed me." I didn't use her idea for a title—*How to Die Laughing*—but it was a good try.

Thanks to my lifelong best friend, Celia Snavely, without whose wisdom, insight, compassion, humor, and love I could not have understood, much less written about, the whole story.

Thanks to my editor, Betsy Thorpe, who helped me to believe I really had something important to say and that I said it well.

Thanks to Kim Matthews, who helped me shape the premise for this book, and to William Rikard, my legal consultant and Harvey's friend, law partner, and fishing buddy.

Thanks to our many friends who have taught us what true

Acknowledgments

friendship really is; to the people who are Covenant Presbyterian Church for their practical and prayerful support; to Harvey's colleagues, who honored him with their companionship and esteem over nearly forty years of a storied career; to so many in the medical community who helped us beyond the call of duty; and to my special widowed friends, who met with me many times, answered my questions, and generously shared their stories.

Thanks to the strangers we met along the way—some mentioned in this book and some not—who offered prayers, hugs, time, kind words, and helping hands throughout our ordeal. You can't go through what we did without realizing just how good people can be.

And to Harvey: I hope you had some idea of just how much you have been loved.

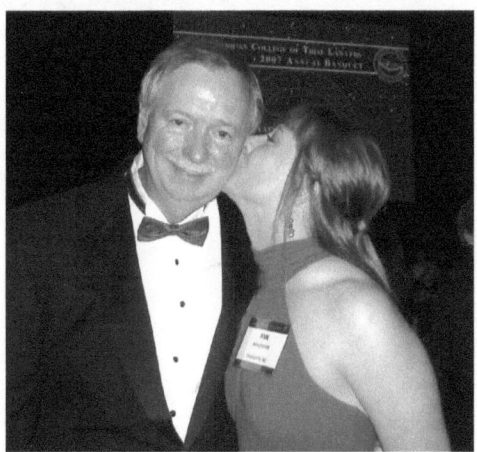

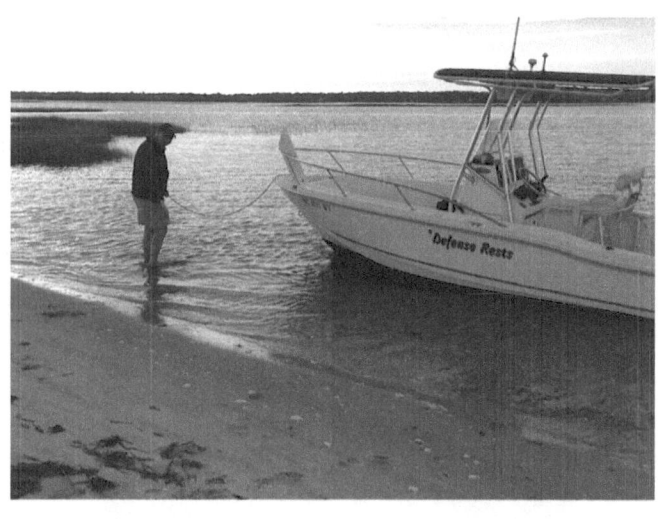

Suggested Reading

Brothers, Dr. Joyce. *Widowed*

Haugk, Kenneth C., PhD. *Don't Sing Songs to a Heavy Heart: How to relate to those who are suffering*

Didion, Joan. *The Year of Magical Thinking*

Fumia, Molly. *Safe Passage: Words to Help the Grieving Hold Fast and Let Go*

Ginsburg, Genevieve Davis, MS. *Widow to Widow (Thoughtful, practical ideas for rebuilding your life)*

Guthrie, Nancy. *What Grieving People Wish You Knew*

Hicks, Josephine. *If There Is Anything I Can Do*

Kessler, David. *Grief.com*, website

Kubler-Ross, Elisabeth and Kessler, David. *On Grief and Grieving*

Lamotte, Anne. *Stitches*

L'Engle, Madeleine. *Two-Part Invention*

Sandberg, Sheryl and Grant, Adam. *When the Worst Happens*

www.ingramcontent.com/pod-product-compliance
Lightning Source LLC
Chambersburg PA
CBHW031055080526
44587CB00011B/691